Protect and Serve

The 7-Day Health Improvement Program Cookbook with Music Medicine for Gut Health, Stress Management, Anxiety and Depression

DENNIS D. BURKHARDT *and* JUDITH PINKERTON

Copyright ©2021 Music 4 Life, Inc. All rights reserved

No part of this book may be reproduced, or stored in a retrieval system, or transmitted in any form or by any means, electronic, mechanical, photocopying, recording, or otherwise, without express written permission of the publisher.

Music 4 Life, Inc.

8465 West Sahara Avenue, #111-244

Las Vegas, NV 89117 USA

themusic4life.com

ISBN 978-0-9745147-3-4

Table of Contents

Chapter 1 1

   Your Gut is Packed With Bacteria (and that's a good thing!)..........1

Chapter 2 5

   What to Expect from an Unhealthy Gut 5

Chapter 3 11

   Potential Causes of an Unhealthy Gut 11

Chapter 4 13

   What is "Leaky Gut Syndrome?" 13

Chapter 5 19

   Elimination - A Food Test 19

Chapter 6 25

   Food Allergies vs. Sensitivities...25

Chapter 7 29

   How Your Gut Responds to Music 29

Chapter 8 33

   10 Strategies to Enhance Gut Health 33

Chapter 9 39

   21 Recipes - Gluten & Dairy free 39

Chapter 10 101

   21 Music & Quotes for Relaxation & Positive Mindset 101

Special Offer 108

References 109

About The Authors 113

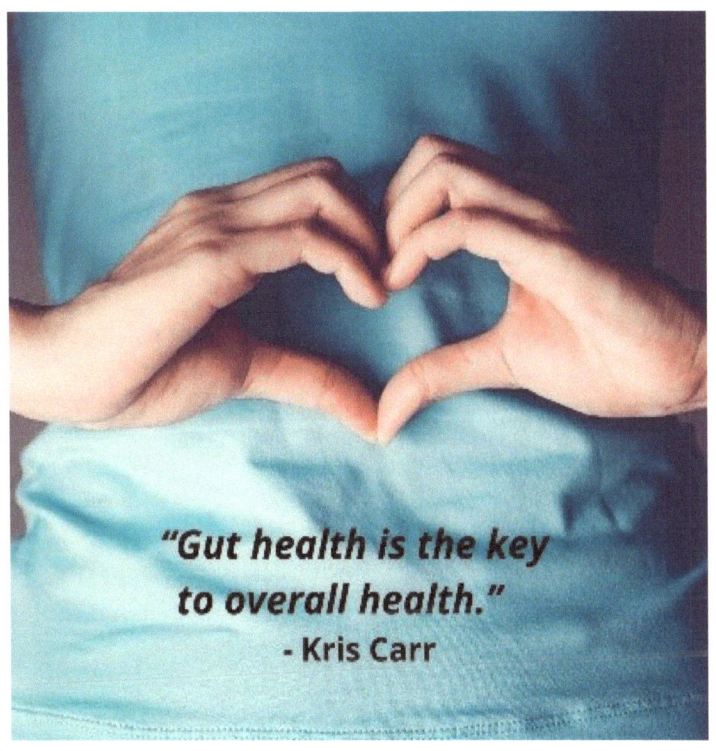

Disclaimer of Medical Advice

You, the reader, are responsible for your own medical care, treatment, and oversight. All content provided within this book does not constitute the provision of medical advice nor does it substitute for independent professional medical judgment, advise, diagnosis, or treatment. Because medical information changes constantly, the information provided in this book may not be current, complete or exhaustive. Therefore, it is recommended that you seek the advice of your qualified health provider, with no delay, regarding your health related to treatment or standard of care.

Introduction by Judith Pinkerton

Most people never consider the importance of gut health. Dennis and I have teamed up to create this 7-Day Gut Stress Program which utilizes 3 healthy strategies to support feeling better. Rather than producing just another cookbook, we decided to share what we have learned from our years in the Chiropractic and Music Medicine fields from a stress perspective. Stress is something we all experience, yet most of us don't fully understand how it impacts our total health.

First we start with gut healthy recipes. These are the recipes from our kitchen that helped me get my gut health under control when life kept throwing me curve balls. When we are not attentive to the needs of our body that one oversight can create a cascade of negative effects.

Second we address stress in your environment. Did you know digestion is affected by stress and may impact which nutrients will be absorbed by the intestines? It can also pave the way for gut bacteria to pass through the intestinal barrier and enter the body which is normally protected from this bacteria. According to the American Psychological Association stress may even be linked with changes in gut bacteria which can influence your mood (APA, 2018).

If you're eating while listening to disturbing news, or arguments or crying children it will create stress which may negatively impact digestion. Included in our program are music listening suggestions to reduce stress and put your mind in a positive space. Over the years friends have marveled at how I remain so positive and happy despite extreme stress from numerous life challenges including cancer. I will share some success tips along the way.

Third, after you've finished your meal, or perhaps while you are cooking it, you can reflect on the carefully selected quotes that are included to support a positive mindset. Positive mindset is key to most success. That's why we've included opportunities for reflection in our program.

There's a lot more going on in your digestive system than just digesting food, absorbing nutrients, and eliminating waste. If your health is less than perfect, your gut is likely to be at least partially to blame! I learned this lesson right after relocating from Anchorage, Alaska to Las Vegas, Nevada. My bloated belly and digestive tract had become impacted: it felt hard as a rock. I met a friend who introduced me to alternative therapies supporting gut health, including colonics, juicing and testing myself for food allergies or sensitivities. The colonic specialist informed me I had a dairy intolerance because my body manufactured too much mucous which created the intestinal impact. So I started investigating what gut health meant. After doing a 10-day test on removing almost everything from my diet and re-introducing food items (read chapter 5), I discovered I had a wheat sensitivity with a large, white, itchy welt magically appearing on my forehead within 6 hours of eating a specific hot cereal.

Stress was a huge factor in my life. At that time I was a new single mom with my 4-year old daughter. I was new to the city and working multiple jobs, including Las Vegas show-symphony-gig violinist, fine jewelry sales at J.C.Penney, healing music presentations, and temp assignments through a business placement agency. Life was really overwhelming, and I needed help.

You know what they say, "be careful what you ask for." Well I prayed for a nanny. But instead I got a knight in shining armor. I met my soulmate. He cared so deeply for me, being attentive to the signs of anything not optimal in my health, and intervened to protect me when needed. Our romance quickened and I was swept off my feet with his caring support, and service of healthy, gourmet meals. He supported my life. We were married within six months of meeting and ten months later we birthed a son into our blended family of 4 children.

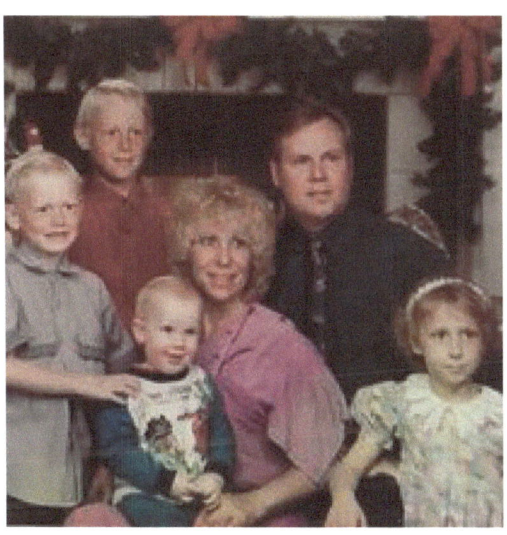

There is a spiritual connection that binds us. Dr. Dennis D. Burkhardt, my soulmate and husband, doubles as my protector – and what a bonus – my chiropractor too! We met through church and he has proven to be my life saver. Our romance has been a harmonic balance of faith, love, children and alternative therapies which are foundational to our marriage.

Not only did I come to realize how vital chiropractic adjustments are to our family's well-being, but his ability to recommend levels of vitamin and mineral supplements was uncanny. My adrenals had become exhausted escalating from one child to four in one year, including a newborn. He replenished my energy with supplements, using his skill as a kinesiologist and general manager of a nutritional manufacturing facility. He was attentive to my dietary discoveries and would instantly provide a food fix with adapted recipes to support my best gut health. These past three decades have been rich with investigations into optimizing our health.

I've learned that the digestive tract is a fascinating combination of activities. Food is being digested. Some of that food is allowed to be absorbed into the bloodstream, while other components of the meal and the digestive process are prevented from crossing over into the body. Think about it. Your digestive tract is a long tube that starts at your mouth and ends at the other end. The stuff that goes into one end and comes out the other never really made it into the body. Water is reabsorbed in the large intestine. The waste continues to travel through. There are also bacteria that play an important role in all of this. Having the proper types and levels of bacteria in the digestive tract make a huge difference in your overall health.

Consider how horrible you feel when your digestive system is out of sorts. Heartburn, cramps, bloating, gas, diarrhea, and constipation are just a few of the common inconveniences of an unhealthy gut. But it goes much deeper than that. There are implications that an unhealthy gut can contribute to diabetes, heart disease, Alzheimer's, and cancer. It pays to have a healthy gut. In this program, we'll look at the signs and symptoms of an unhealthy gut and discuss ways to bring an unhealthy gut back to a state of good health.

Consider information in Chapters 1-8 as a way to learn more about the importance of good gut health. Chapters 9-10 will provide opportunities to change the way you eat, think and feel.

Chapter 1: Your Gut is Packed With Bacteria. You have more bacterial cells in your body than you do human cells. Maybe what we consider to be a human body is really a bacterial organism surrounded by human cells.

Chapter 2: What to Expect from an Unhealthy Gut. An unhealthy gut can cause more than digestive tract discomfort. An unhealthy gut can be the primary cause of many life-threatening diseases.

Chapter 3: Potential Causes of an Unhealthy Gut. By now you know that an unhealthy gut is a serious matter. Now, you're going to find out what creates an unhealthy gut.

Chapter 4: What is "Leaky Gut Syndrome"? There is disagreement between the medical community and alternative health communities about the existence and effects of leaky gut syndrome because the gut is still largely a mystery. But it's worth considering if Leaky Gut Syndrome could be a serious issue with serious health implications for you.

Chapter 5: Elimination – A Food Test. An elimination plan is something that everyone should do at least every few years. It's one of the most life-altering things a person can do for themselves.

Chapter 6: Food Allergies vs Sensitivities. Poor gut health can contribute to these serious issues.

Chapter 7: How Your Gut Responds to Music. Reducing stress can strengthen your immune system and play an important role in gut health. Music may be your best medicine.

Chapter 8: 10 Strategies to Enhance Gut Health. What can you do to boost your gut health? You will find suggestions here for both men and women!

Chapter 9: 21 Recipes – Gluten & Dairy Free. These gluten free and dairy free meals have been tested over time as delicious and healthy for the gut for those of us that have those allergies or sensitivities! Get your food fix!

Chapter 10: 21 Music & Quotes for Relaxation & Positive Mindset. Selected to enhance relaxation and support a positive mindset, twenty-one music selections and matching quotes are excerpted from my new program "Power Up Your Life with Music." This 365-day program delivers a series of daily inspirations and matching music from my music therapy practice which embraces alternative therapies. Find tips and a special offer in this book to unlock stress management strategies for gaining control over the debilitating effects of anxiety and depression.

✳✳✳

My hope: these recipe gems and mindset treasures become rich enhancements for the lives of both men and women as Dennis and I seek to protect and serve you.

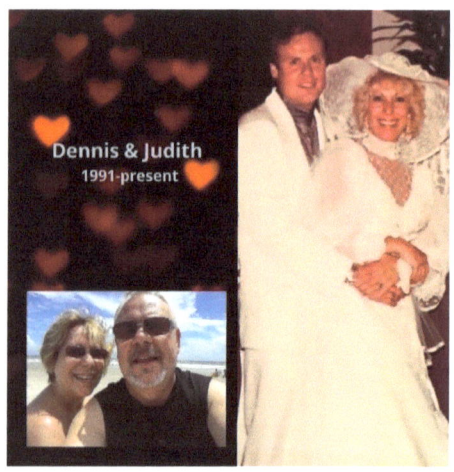

"I think that age as a number is not nearly as important as health. You can be in poor health and be pretty miserable at 40 or 50. If you're in good health, you can enjoy things into your 80s."

- BOB BARKER

Chapter 1

Your Gut is Packed With Bacteria (and that's a good thing!)

Your gut is rich with bacteria. In fact, over 100 trillion bacteria can be found in the gut. These include both good and bad bacteria. This collection of bacteria is referred to as the gut microbiota or gut microbiome. Some of these bacteria, such as E. Coli, can cause disease. However, most of the bacteria in your body are there to help ("Can Gut Bacteria Improve Your Health?," 2016).

They are an important component of your immune system and help to maintain balance in your body. There are a few hundred types of bacteria in the human gut that have a variety of effects on the human body.

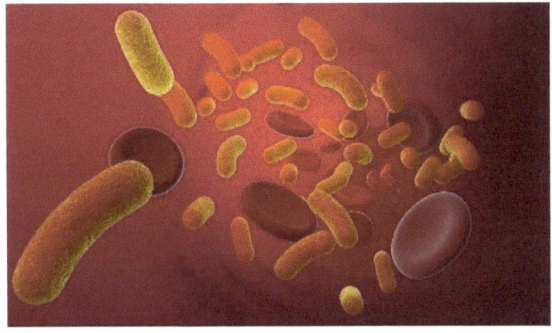

For example, there are bacteria that increase inflammation, while others decrease it. Other bacteria aid with digestion and the absorption of nutrients. Scientists are still discovering all the various ways these bacteria influence the various systems of the body. If the ratio of these bacteria becomes unbalanced, it negatively affects your health.

Consider that nearly 70% of the immune system is managed by the gut ("5 Ways To Boost Your Immune System Through Your Gut," n.d.). There are also over 100 million neurons in the gut that can communicate with other cells and organs in the body (Underwood, 2018).

Many health conditions are believed to be either caused or influenced by poor gut health (Zhang et al., 2015; Stone, 2020; Torgan, 2013; University of Zurich, 2018; Hitti, 2004; Clapp et al., 2017; Alkasir, 2017).

Some of these include:

- Type 2 diabetes
- Heart disease
- Skin and hair issues
- Cancer
- Rheumatoid arthritis
- Multiple sclerosis
- Asthma
- Allergies
- Anxiety
- Depression

- Dementia

- Obesity

- Inflammatory bowel disease

If the bacteria in your gut are out of balance, you're suffering more than necessary. Many of the health challenges you might be facing could be significantly helped by creating a healthier gut. A healthy gut has the right types of bacteria in the proper ratios.

Chapter 2

What to Expect from an Unhealthy Gut

There are three primary consequences of an unhealthy gut: inflammation, nutrient absorption issues, and immune / autoimmune issues (Dix, 2020). All of these issues can have devastating health consequences, including anxiety and depression.

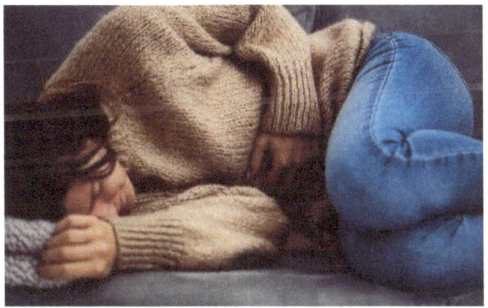

Inflammation

It is believed that the gut is the primary cause of inflammation in the body. Inflammation is a primary contributor to disease and also results in many uncomfortable symptoms. An inflamed body is an uncomfortable body. There are several symptoms that can be caused by inflammation, including:

1. Insomnia. It might be hard to believe, but gut inflammation has been shown to be a cause of insomnia. If you have trouble

sleeping, and you're unable to pinpoint another cause, your sleepless nights might be due to gut inflammation.

2. Acne and other skin disorders. It is believed that acne, psoriasis, and many other skin conditions can be caused by inflammation in the digestive tract.

3. Depression. Inflammation that reaches the brain can influence the production and ratio of neurotransmitters.

4. Anxiety. Anxiety without an identifiable cause can also be caused by inflammation.

5. Fatigue. Inflammation can lead to imbalances in the body's stress hormones, resulting in adrenal fatigue and overall fatigue throughout the body.

6. Brain fog. Inflammation in the brain can be a cause of brain fog.

7. Hormone imbalances. In females, gut inflammation can alter the levels of hormones and cause hot flashes, alter menstrual cycle length, and affect PMS symptoms. In men, hormonal imbalances due to gut inflammation can result in fatigue, muscle loss, erectile dysfunction, and poor memory.

8. Thyroid-related symptoms. Systemic inflammation in the body can make it more challenging for your body to utilize thyroid hormone properly. This can result in symptoms of hypothyroidism, even if your thyroid hormone levels are normal.

Nutrient Absorption Issues

The nutrients that your body are able to absorb and utilize are affected by your gut bacteria. While most of the absorption of nutrients in the human body occurs in the small intestine, there is also a significant amount of digestion that occurs in the large intestine.

Nearly all of the digestion that occurs in the large intestine is the result of bacterial activity. The bacteria ferment the remaining proteins and carbohydrates that made it beyond the small intestine. These proteins and carbohydrates are converted into short-chain fatty acids which can be used for energy in the body.

Bacteria in the gut are also needed to synthesize vitamin B12, thiamin, folate, riboflavin, vitamin K, and biotin. A healthy gut calls for an anti-inflammatory diet necessary for synthesis and absorption of nutrients.

Autoimmune and Immune-Related Issues

Interestingly, gut bacteria are believed to play a huge role in autoimmune diseases. It turns out that proteins produced by common gut bacteria can serve as the trigger for many autoimmune diseases such as ulcerative colitis and rheumatoid arthritis. These proteins mimic proteins that naturally occur in the human body. The immune system becomes sensitized to these proteins and begins attacking these proteins and the naturally occurring proteins.

Leaky gut syndrome can also contribute to autoimmune disorders. We'll discuss leaky gut syndrome shortly.

An unhealthy gut can be the primary cause of these eight autoimmune disorders.

1. Celiac disease. Celiac disease is an immune disorder that prevents people from eating gluten without injury to the small intestine. The immune system is activated in the presence of gluten and attacks the small intestine.

2. Gluten intolerance. There are many people that don't have a true gluten allergy but are very sensitive to gluten in the diet.

3. Inflammatory bowel disease. This is a broad term that describes disorders that involve chronic inflammation in the digestive tract. It includes several diseases, the most common of which are ulcerative colitis and Crohn's disease.

4. Depression. There is mounting evidence that an autoimmune issue is at least partially responsible for some cases of depression.

5. Irritable bowel syndrome. While celiac disease affects the small intestine, irritable bowel syndrome targets the large intestine. Irritable bowel syndrome doesn't cause permanent damage but can be troubling to manage. An immune system response or changes in gut bacteria are often to blame.

6. Food allergies and reactivity. Bacteria imbalances in the gut have been implicated in many food allergy cases. Intolerances to certain foods can also be blamed on gut flora.

7. Joint pain. Rheumatoid arthritis can cause great joint pain and long-term damage in the joints that are affected. This is an autoimmune disease that affects 1.5 million people in the

United States ("Arthritis by the Numbers," 2019).

8. Hypothyroidism. The most common cause of hypothyroidism is an autoimmune disease that is often treated by addressing infections in the gut.

- Autoimmune diseases can be debilitating and life threatening.

- 100 trillion bacteria have the potential to either cause a lot of challenges or to support good health.

Hopefully, it's beginning to become clear just how important a healthy gut is for general health.

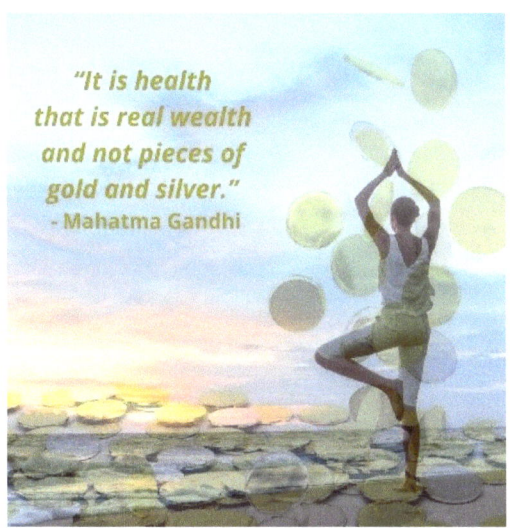

Chapter 3

Potential Causes of an Unhealthy Gut

What causes an unhealthy gut? There are many causes, and it's likely that researchers will find more in the next few years. Fortunately, the causes of an unhealthy gut can be largely eliminated by making wise decisions about what you eat. Smart choices at the dining room table can go a long way toward creating a healthy digestive system. Consider eliminating the following six causes of an unhealthy gut from your life.

1. Unhealthy diet. A healthy diet is specific to the person. A diet that boosts gut health is one that supports the good bacteria in the body, doesn't upset the digestive tract, provides the proper amount of calories and nutrients, and is sustainable. Food allergies and sensitivities are also important considerations.

2. The wrong balance of bacteria. This is primarily a function of diet.

3. Alcohol. Alcohol can disrupt the digestive process and also impact the natural balance of bacteria in the gut.

4. Anxiety and Stress. There are studies that show that anxiety and stress can impact gut health. Not only are the gut bacteria affected, but food consumption and digestion are also impacted. You might feel compelled to overeat or to eat poorly when stressed. Or perhaps you find it challenging to eat when stressed.

Anxiety and stress can also contribute to heartburn, nausea, diarrhea, and constipation, and also reduce sleep quality.

5. Poor blood sugar control. Does insulin resistance disrupt the bacteria in the gut, or do the bacteria in the gut create insulin resistance? Actually, both situations occur.

6. Antibiotics. Healthy bacteria are killed in the gut with antibiotics which have a broad spectrum of action, including diarrhea.

As with many other health-related issues, diet is a primary cause of an unhealthy gut. A healthy diet is one of the best ways to boost your general health and your gut health. Most of the causes of an unhealthy gut can be minimized by making smart food choices which considers an anti-inflammatory diet that is gluten free and dairy free if you have those sensitivities or allergies.

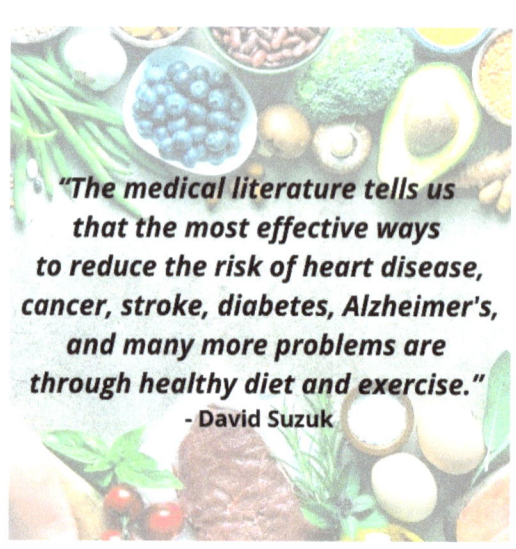

Chapter 4

What is Leaky Gut Syndrome?

The lining of the small intestine is very important to good health. It provides a barrier between the bloodstream and the contents of the intestine.

Not everything that enters or lives in the intestine should enter the bloodstream. It is up to the cells of the intestinal lining to make this important decision. In a healthy gastrointestinal tract, nothing is able to enter the bloodstream without the blessing of these cells lining the gut wall. This is a healthy function of our bodies and is referred to as Intestinal Permeability. The scientific phenomenon of the gut increasing in permeability is referred to as "leaky gut." Disagreement exists between many in the medical and alternative health and nutrition communities on the existence and consequence of what is termed "Leaky Gut Syndrome." According to these alternative health practitioners and some nutritionists, leaky gut syndrome is the result of the intestinal lining not being 100% intact and undesirable substances entering the blood through the intestine (Gundry, 2018; McMillen, n.d.).

According to this alternative school of thought these substances can wreak havoc in the body four ways.

1. The liver is overburdened. When toxic substances enter the body, the liver is tasked with eliminating those substances. You can't live without your liver, so reducing its workload as much

as possible is a good idea.

2. The immune system is activated. A foreign substance in the body can stimulate an immune response. Unnecessary immune activity can be damaging to the human body.

3. Inflammation occurs. Immune system activity can trigger inflammation. Inflammation is believed to be the cause of many serious diseases.

4. Increased likelihood of food allergies and sensitivities. Leaky gut syndrome is one pathway that can create food allergies and sensitivities.

Symptoms of "Leaky Gut Syndrome"

There are a wide variety of symptoms, which are believed to be the result of "leaky gut syndrome" that can make it challenging to identify the cause with a high degree of certainty. These symptoms include:

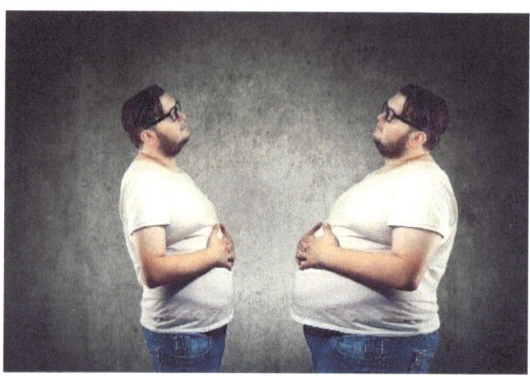

- Regular bouts of a bloated belly, diarrhea, gas, constipation, or digestive-related pain

- Asthma

- Seasonal allergies

- Rashes or other skin-related issues

- Multiple food sensitivities

- Auto-immune disorders such as lupus and rheumatoid arthritis

- Brain fog

- Poor memory

- Headaches

- Fatigue

- Anxiety, depression

- Difficulty concentrating

This is a pretty wide-ranging list of symptoms! If you have one or more of these symptoms, might you have leaky gut syndrome?

Maybe.

Let's consider what contributes to leaky gut syndrome.

Causes of Leaky Gut

Most experts are in agreement that a leaky gut can have several contributing causes, including:

- Stress

- Toxins and infections

- Food selection

What these factors have in common is that they create inflammation which many consider to be the primary cause of leaky gut syndrome.

The primary strategy for combating leaky gut syndrome is believed to involve removing these sources of inflammation.

Stress

Chronic stress is believed to be a significant contributor to leaky gut syndrome. Stress may lead to inflammation. Stress may also inhibit the immune response which permits various sources of inflammation to go unchecked.

The best ways to eliminate this contributing factor are to learn and practice relaxation techniques and to minimize the amount of stress in your life (Fraser, 2018; Ariciu, n.d.).

Toxins and Infections

The bacteria that normally occur in the gut can grow excessively under the right conditions and cause damage to the intestinal lining. Parasites are another type of infection that can damage the intestine.

These bacteria can create a variety of toxins and enzymes that corrupt the lining of the intestine and interfere with normal digestion.

Food Selection

Diet is considered to play the largest role in causing leaky gut. There are several foods commonly considered to be problematic:

- Refined grains
- Refined sugars
- Artificial colorings
- Artificial flavorings
- Preservatives
- Processed foods
- Foods that result in sensitivities or stimulate the immune system. These foods vary from person to person.

The human body in general, and the immune system specifically, don't reliably recognize these substances as foods. These substances can lead to immune system activity, burden the liver, and cause inflammation.

Some people are very sensitive to certain foods. One simple way to identify these foods is to do an elimination diet as the first step in creating an anti-inflammatory diet.

Chapter 5

Elimination - A Food Test

I was miserable, and I didn't understand why. My stomach was bloated and hard as a rock. And it certainly wasn't a six pack from working out! (Whisper: I was severely constipated.) I researched to try to understand the cause of my misery and settled on trying the elimination diet.

The revelations came quickly and I discovered I had sensitivities and allergies to certain foods. For example, a four inch long white itchy welt appeared on my forehead within hours of re-introducing a wheat-based hot cereal into my diet. Pasta (also containing wheat) seemed to harden, almost like cement, in my digestive tract. You'll never guess what I noticed about sugar. When I brought it back into my diet, my neck muscles stiffened, really?! Dairy consumption was accompanied by nausea and an overly abundant supply of mucous, YUK! This exercise was so easy to do. I wish I had discovered it years ago. It has proven to be one of the most valuable things I have done for my health and comfort.

- Judith Pinkerton

Since the food you consume can have such an impact on your overall health and your gut health, finding the foods that don't agree with your body can be a powerful tool for enhancing your health. An elimination diet is an experiment of sorts. It will help you to identify the specific foods that cause negative symptoms when ingested. In a nutshell, you eliminate all suspect foods in your diet, and then add them back one at a time. The offending foods are easy to identify with this method. There are two parts to all elimination diets:

1. Elimination

2. Reintroduction

Elimination Phase

In the elimination phase, the goal is to eliminate all the foods that could possibly be causing a negative reaction. It's important to avoid all of these possible irritating foods during this phase. And of course it is important to consult your doctor prior to beginning any new dietary process.

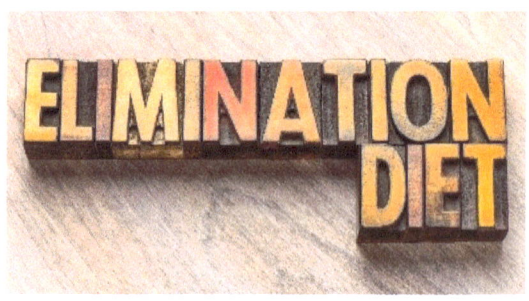

You can make your own list of foods to avoid, but the most common culprits include:

- Dairy

- Eggs

- Shellfish

- Soy
- Citrus
- Sugar
- Gluten/wheat
- Artificial colors
- Preservatives
- Artificial sweeteners
- Preservatives
- Nuts

It might seem like there's nothing left to eat, but that's not true. In fact, most of the naturally occurring foods are still available to you, such as:

- Unprocessed meat and fish
- Beans, rice, lentils
- Vegetables
- Non-citrus fruit

This is probably the way your mother always wanted you to eat anyway!

How long does the elimination phase take? Two to three weeks is suggested. That's enough time for your body to stabilize and reach a baseline state.

Before and after the elimination phase, it's important to evaluate yourself. Use any rating scale you like (i.e. A to D, 1-10, 1-5 stars, it's up you) and create a chart to rate yourself on the following items before you start and after you are done:

- Sleep quality
- Focus
- Mood
- Physical pain - headaches, joint pain, muscle pain
- Anxiety
- Digestion - stomach pain, bowel habits, bloated belly
- Energy
- Skin quality / blemishes

Now that you have established your experience of those items before and after the elimination phase, it's time to begin reintroducing foods.

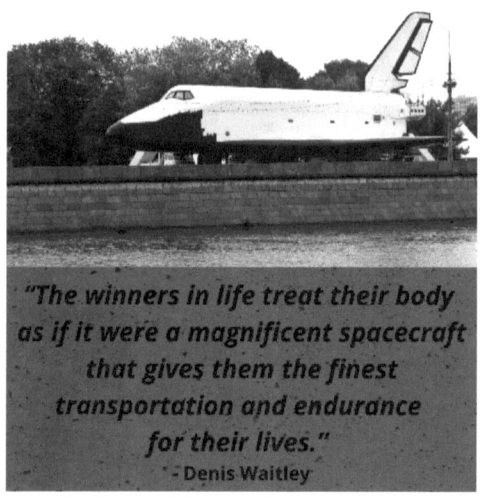

Reintroduction Phase

First, notice how you feel. Most people find that they feel better than they have in a long time. Most of us eat a lot of things our bodies don't appreciate. It seems that the most enticing foods are rarely the foods that maximize our health.

Now it's time to discover which foods you should be avoiding on a permanent basis. You might be surprised by what you find. And, you'll be glad that you committed to performing this experiment on yourself.

The reintroduction phase is when things become interesting. Follow this 5-step process to reintroduce foods back into your diet.

1. Choose one food you avoided. Add it back into your diet. Eat this food a couple of times each day for 1-3 days.

2. Re-evaluate how you feel. Rate yourself on the same items you considered before and after the elimination phase.

3. Note any changes. If your ratings went down, you know that you should avoid that food in the future. If you don't notice any changes, that food can be considered safe to eat.

4. Go back and reintroduce another food. Only add one food at a time. If you add more than one food and feel worse, how will you know which food is causing negative issues?

5. Keep experimenting. You might find that certain nuts are fine, but others are not. Maybe you handle one artificial sweetener but not the others. Be logical and perform the necessary experiments to narrow down the list of foods that might be causing challenges.

This won't take as long as you might think. You probably don't eat as many different foods as you think you do. In a relatively short amount of time, you can gain knowledge about the foods you eat that can change your life. Eat smarter.

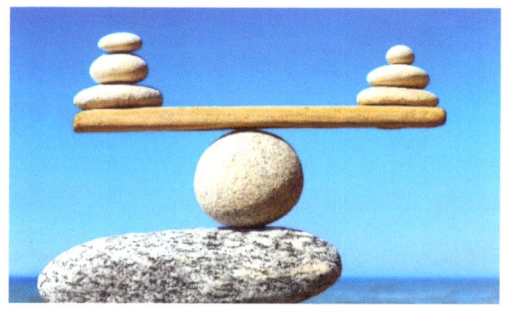

*"If we could give every individual the right
amount of nourishment and exercise,
not too little and not too much,
we would have found
the safest way to health."*
- Hippocrates

Chapter 6

Food Allergies vs. Sensitivities

There is part of the population that has one or more food allergies. And there are far more people that suffer from food sensitivities. Many people claim to be allergic to a food group, when they really have a food sensitivity.

So what is the difference? Mainly, it is the involvement of the immune system.

For example, there are people that are lactose intolerant. When they consume milk products that haven't had the lactose removed, they experience significant gas, bloating, cramps, and diarrhea. However, this isn't a true allergy. They simply lack the enzyme to digest lactose.

The bacteria in the colon feast on the lactose which would have been previously absorbed by someone that was not lactose intolerant. All of the gas and other side effects are produced by these bacteria.

A true food allergy includes an immune response. It's as if the body views the food as a foreign invader. Antibodies are released by the body to attack the food. The inflammatory response can be quite severe.

Food allergy symptoms include:

- Hives

- Itchiness

- Swelling of throat, tongue, face, or lips

- Abdominal pain

- Nausea, vomiting, diarrhea

- Dizziness or fainting

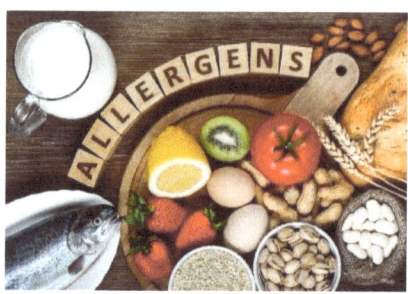

In extreme situations, allergic reactions to food can even be life-threatening. There are just a handful of foods responsible for 90% of all food allergies. These are peanuts, milk, soy, eggs, wheat, fish, tree nuts, and shellfish.

Approximately 10.8% of the population actually suffer from one or more food allergies, whereas 19% believe they have a food allergy (Gupta et al., 2019).

Food sensitivities, or intolerance, are much more common. Most people have at least one food that leaves them feeling worse after they ate it than they did before eating it.

Food sensitivity symptoms include:

- Anxiety

- Irritability

- Fatigue

- Mental fog

- Heartburn, nausea, vomiting, stomach pain, bloated belly, diarrhea

- Headaches

Food allergies are certainly more serious, but food sensitivities can be quite miserable, too. You might be shocked by how much better you feel simply by avoiding all of the foods that don't agree with your body.

You may be able to determine which foods to avoid with the Elimination - A Food Test process. If you feel like you're still having issues with some foods, talk with your doctor. Nowadays, they can determine most foods that cause a negative reaction within your body with a simple skin or blood test.

If you believe you have food allergies, ask your doctor for help pinpointing them. An allergy test will likely provide valuable information that may be difficult to determine with only the Elimination - a Food Test process.

Chapter 7

How Your Gut Responds to Music

Stress has a significant negative impact on your gut. When you experience an increase in nervous tension it causes the acid-producing cells in the wall of your stomach to manufacture more hydrochloric acid. Mix this with excess air and painful intestinal distension occurs. Chronic stress can have an even more serious impact on your gut, even affecting your immune system function.

One Mother told me that on the rare occasions that she had to raise her voice to get her daughter's attention on getting to school on time that she would come home sick with a tummy ache later. Soon after this realization she started playing and singing Barry Manilow's song, "Can't Smile Without You," every day on the ride to school, to eliminate sound-related gut stress. If a temporary change in the sound of a familiar voice can be so disruptive that it causes stomach pain, imagine how powerfully the quality of sound and music can affect our perception and physical experience.

- Judith Pinkerton

Researchers at the University of Oxford believe that we find it difficult to keep our experiences isolated. Their study, published in the "Appetite" journal, gave 116 volunteers small squares of dark chocolate with either 81% or 71% cocoa. They were asked to taste the same chocolate and report on the taste they either ate in silence, or while music was playing. When listening to dissonant staccato notes from a violin they described the chocolate as rough or bitter. But while listening to long legato notes from a flute, participants responded that the chocolate tasted creamier (Carvalho et al., 2017).

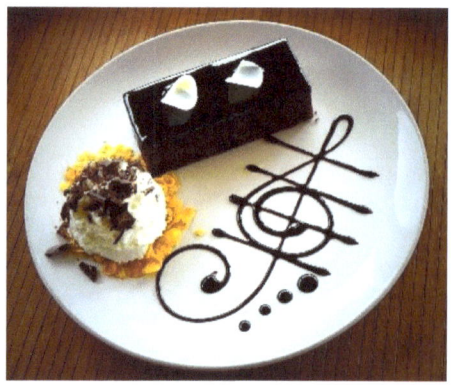

This was validated in another study using Gelato and various types of sound. More relaxing sounds were positively correlated with the perception of sweetness and smoothness, while more intense sound was positively correlated with the perception of bitterness (Lin et al., 2019).

Do you think our music and sound choices affect perceptions of our lives?

Movie Magic Test

Try this quick test at home. While watching a scary movie, notice if you feel tension in your stomach or chest. When it gets to the scariest part turn off the movie sound while continuing to watch.
Does your perception of what's happening in the movie change?
Does it seem more or less scary?
Do you feel tension in your stomach with the sound off? What about when it is on?

Music can impact our tension and stress. The use of music-making for reducing stress and improving mood has been demonstrated in numerous research studies including studies that involve a drumming protocol (Bittman et al., 2001, 2003). So typical relaxation music may not always be the best option for reducing stress. Music listening is a helpful tool for addressing stress and interestingly, music listening can affect our appetite.

The expansive effects music has on our mind and body are amazing. So I decided to investigate the potential effects of music while we eat. I discovered a study of 78 college students who recorded their food intake, meal duration, meal location, time of day and music conditions (i.e. tempo, volume). This was done for a week. There were several environmental factors that influenced food and fluid intake including music listening. Turns out, when they listened to music they also ate more food, drank more fluid and enjoyed longer meal duration as well (Stroebele & de Castro, 2006; Chaput et al., 2011).

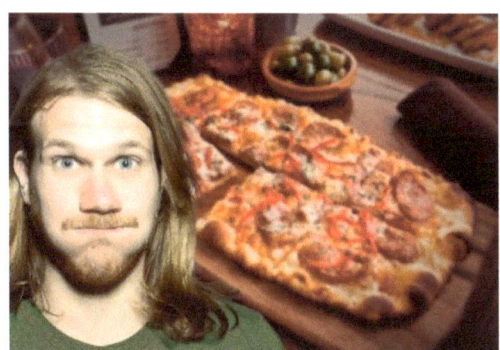

Perhaps college students eating more isn't necessarily a great thing for their health. But consider this in the context of aging. One pervasive problem with many people as they age is that a lack of appetite causes significant weight loss and reduction in energy which may lead to a dangerous falls for people with more brittle bones.

Listening to music can be very pleasant and motivating. But for myself and my clinical clients as a music therapist, I go beyond just listening to music they like.

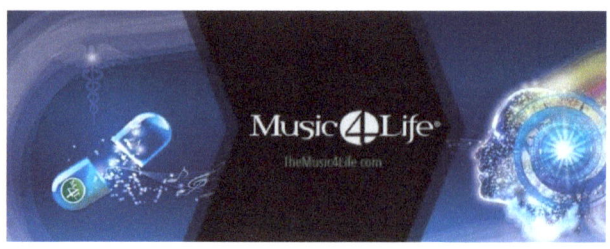

I developed the Music 4 Life® Music Medicine Protocol over the course of 30 years of experience as a professional violinist and as a music therapist. This protocol involves music therapy innovation and Mood Sequence Formulas™. Together, we identify music that moves you emotionally. And then we prescribe a specific music playlist to help you achieve your goals by using the music to move you from unhealthy or unproductive mood states to more productive moods. This allows you to exercise emotions in a very healthy way as you listen.

I do this personally to not only reduce gut stress, but to change my whole perspective on life. I've helped people create prescriptive playlists to support life recovery from destructive habits, to help people transition through grief much more quickly, and to transition out of destructive mood states. If you would like to learn more about this technique visit: themusic4life.com.

- Judith Pinkerton

Chapter 8

10 Strategies to Enhance Gut Health

You understand the value of good gut health, but what can you do to boost the health of your gut? Actually, there's a lot you can do. Thankfully, much of it is quite simple and easy. A few simple changes in your lifestyle can deliver big results.

In addition to the ten strategies listed in this chapter, my stress-reduction preferences include focusing on a positive mindset and listening to music - but not just any music. I use my Music 4 Life® Music Medicine Protocol to keep myself centered, physically and emotionally flexible and mentally optimistic. The result for me has been developing emotional fluidity. 99% of the time, I can stay emotionally and mentally flexible and optimistic, no matter what! REALLY! In addition to the ten strategies listed below, check out Chapter 10 to find some of my favorite life-affirming quotes and motivating music!

- Judith Pinkerton

Enhance gut health with ten activities

1. Eat a natural diet. The only animals on the planet that eat processed foods are humans and the animals that humans feed. Processed foods are unnatural, and we were never intended to eat them. Eat smarter.

2. Ensure that you consume enough fiber. It's not necessary to eat huge amounts of fiber but be sure to meet the recommendations. The numbers vary with gender and age but can be easily found online.

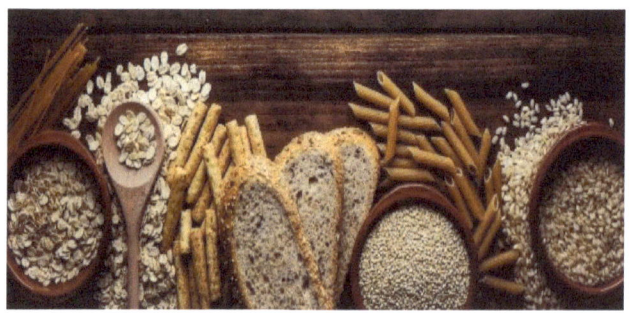

Fiber keeps moving things along in the digestive tract, and soluble fiber is used for food by many of the beneficial bacteria in the gut. High fiber foods include: beans, lentils, artichoke, pears, soybeans, broccoli, avocado, apples, prunes, and many seeds. Eat smarter.

3. Chew well. Well-chewed food makes fewer demands on the digestive system. It requires a lot of work to digest large pieces of food. The digestive process is much more efficient when food is chewed thoroughly.

My mother tells me I've always been a slow eater, so I naturally have been doing this my whole life - yeah!

- Judith

4. Eat fermented foods. Yogurt, miso, kimchi, kefir, tempeh, sauerkraut, and pickles are just a few examples of foods that can boost gut health. Eating at least one of these foods each day can do wonders.

> *I've always had a sensitivity with dairy and do not prefer fermented food. Learning about this strategy motivates me to consume soy yogurt more often.*
>
> *- Judith*

5. Take probiotics. Probiotics add good bacteria to your gut and help to kill off many of the bad bacteria. Be sure to start slowly with the dosing.

   > *When partnering with Dennis to write this book, I was forced to dive into current gut health information which now motivates me to be more intentional with taking non-dairy probiotics. For instance, for me personally I have noticed, if I choose to have alcohol, consuming probiotics the next day is best for me to maintain optimal gut health. There are many probiotic choices out there. Check with your doctor for advice.*
   >
   > *- Judith*

6. Drink plenty of water. Water is used throughout the body. It helps to digest food. It's used in the production of digesting enzymes. It's not necessary to drink a gallon of water each day, but drink according to thirst. Prioritize the consumption of water over other beverages.

   > *Living in the desert for three decades you would think I would be a natural at consuming enough water. I'm not. What I do know is that my lips, face and gut feel good when I am hydrated, so I intentionally set periodic alarms in my cell phone as reminders to drink water now.*
   >
   > *- Judith*

7. Exercise. Exercise is good for every part of your body. Regular movement is also good for helping to move food through the digestive tract and maintain regularity.

   Over the past year, I decided to enlist a personal trainer who customizes my anaerobic workouts and modifies them monthly. I feel so much stronger, energetic, clear-headed, and focused!

   - Judith

8. Get enough sleep. All aspects of health are boosted by sufficient sleep and rest. Your gut health is no different.

   I still struggle with a consistent 7-8 hour sleep regimen. My workaholic, entrepreneurial, life-long focus seems to require a stream of quiet, consecutive hours to produce significant, meaningful new content. I'm much more intentional though with getting better sleep. It definitely makes a difference in all areas of my life when I am well rested.

   - Judith

9. Avoid excess sugar. Sugar throws off the balance of bacteria in the gut. And sugar is unhealthy in general. Eat smarter.

   When I did the Elimination - Food Test process, I discovered sugar made my neck more stiff which is not best for playing the violin or enabling relaxation.

   - Judith

10. Relax. Stress kills. It's bad for your gut, digestion, and overall health. Learn how to relax. It's a learnable skill.

For me, my family and thousands of clients, the Music 4 Life® Music Medicine Protocol works best in letting go of tension, anxiety, anger, depression or sadness to experience deeper relaxation.

- Judith

Can you see that these are all behaviors that are under your control? One of the best ways to enhance your health is to strengthen the health of your gut. These 10 items can go a long way toward that goal.

Conclusion

Scientists and the medical community are only beginning to understand the vast influence that the gut has on the rest of the body. The immune system and the nervous system are heavily influenced by gut health.

The bacteria naturally found in the gut play a pivotal role in both health and disease. Heart disease, autoimmune diseases, neurological diseases, and many other states of poor health are believed to be at least partially caused by the bacteria found in the gut.

Stress also has an impact on how your gut responds. Using prescriptive music listening to modulate your mood may have a significant positive effect on not only your gut, but your happiness and well-being overall.

Gut health can be heavily influenced by the food choices you make each day: avoid foods that disagree with your body to enhance your health. Eat smarter.

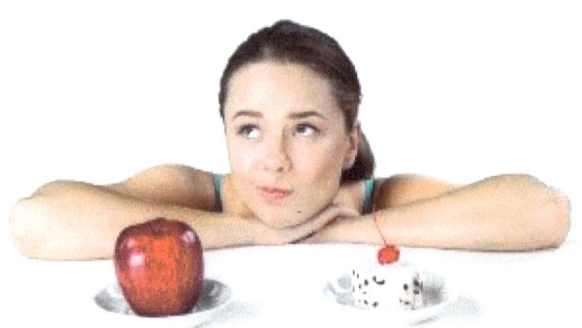

Chapter 9

21 Recipes - Gluten & Dairy free

Although I don't have gut problems with gluten and dairy, as a chiropractor, I focus on optimal health for my wife of 30 years, along with family and friends benefiting too. And they inspire me to share these recipes with you for your "food fix." Incorporate them into your life along with the gut health information from prior chapters, and you may be surprised that current health issues transform in record time. Mix and match the meals to your liking as the daily order is not a prescriptive sequence. Start aiding your healthy gut now: make these yummy recipes I've created or adapted especially for Judith!

- Dennis D. Burkhardt, D.C.

7 Breakfasts

Day 1 Granola Cereal Gluten Free

Day 2 Instant Pot Yogurt Lactose Free

Day 3 Instant Pot Steel Cut Oats

Day 4 Eggs Benedict with Hollandaise Sauce Gluten & Dairy Free

Day 5 Mango Kale Smoothie with Banana Nut Bread Gluten & Dairy Free

Day 6 Biscuits and Gravy Gluten & Dairy Free

Day 7 Overnight French Toast Gluten Free

7 Lunches

Day 1 Cowboy Caviar Gluten & Dairy Free

Day 2 Tortilla Soup

Day 3 Butternut Squash Soup

Day 4 Keto Lettuce Wraps

Day 5 Chili with Cornbread Egg, Gluten & Dairy Free

Day 6 Keto Zucchini Ravioli

Day 7 Fish Sticks Gluten Free

7 Dinners

Day 1 Shipwreck Stew

Day 2 Keto Beef & Broccoli

Day 3 Keto Creamy Tuscan Chicken

Day 4 Keto Instant Pot Ribs

Day 5 Instant Pot Dal

Day 6 Pasta e Fagioli Soup Gluten Free

Day 7 Keto Asian Cabbage Stir Fry

At the end of each recipe is Judith's recommended music and related quote to support a positive mindset while cooking and eating.

Day 1 Breakfast

Granola Cereal Gluten Free

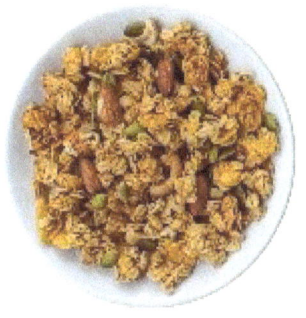

Serving size: 6-8

Ingredients:

- 1 cup hazelnuts
- 1 cup almonds
- 1 cup pecans
- 1/3 cup pumpkin seeds
- 1/3 cup sunflower seeds
- 6 tbsp sweetener of choice (I use brown coconut sugar)
- 1/2 cup flaxseed meal/powder

- 1 large egg White
- 1/4 cup butter or ghee * 1 tsp vanilla extract

Directions:

1. Preheat oven to 325 degrees.
2. Chop nuts individually in a blender or food processor to the consistency you would like.
3. Chop pumpkin seeds & sunflower seeds for only several seconds.
4. Put everything back in the food processor and blend.
5. Add sweetener, flaxseed, egg butter and vanilla. Pulse until well mixed, but do not over pulse.
6. Line 9 x 13 baking sheet with parchment paper and put mixture on the baking sheet.
7. Bake for 15-18 minutes.
8. Remove from the oven and let cool before storing in an airtight container.
9. Eat by itself or with homemade yogurt (reference Day 2 Breakfast) with fruit.

My mother-in-law Carol introduced me to this yummy recipe which has become a staple in my diet. Thank you, Carol!

✳✳✳

Music: "Psyche" by Chris Spheeris

"We can only appreciate the miracle of a sunrise if we have waited in the darkness."

- Sapra Reddy

✳✳✳

Day 1 Lunch

Cowboy Caviar Gluten & Dairy Free

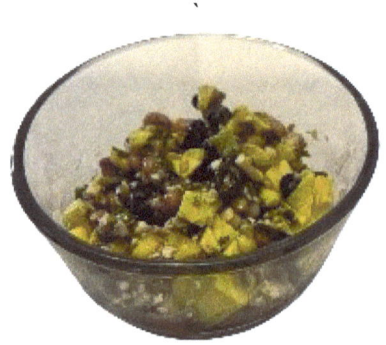

Serving size: 8-10

Ingredients:

- 2 cups frozen corn
- 1 can black eyed peas, drained
- 2 cups dairy free pepper jack cheese
- 1 bunch cilantro, chopped
- 1 can black beans, drained
- 2 avocados, diced
- 1 bunch green onions, chopped

Dressing:

- 1/3 cup olive oil
- 2 tbsp of garlic
- 1/3 cup red wine vinegar

Directions:

1. Mix dressing and pour over ingredients, then mix thoroughly.
2. Best to marinate 24 hours, but can be eaten earlier.
3. Eat with gluten free pita or corn chips.

Our dear friends Alyssa and Sharon introduced this to Judith during a retreat in their beautiful home, and as you can imagine I was tasked with duplicating this yummy recipe immediately upon her return! Thank you, Alyssa and Sharon!

✸✸✸

Music: "Feeling Good" by Michael Buble

"As you think thoughts that feel good to you, you will be in harmony with who you really are."

- Abraham Hicks

✸✸✸

Day 1 Dinner

Shipwreck Stew

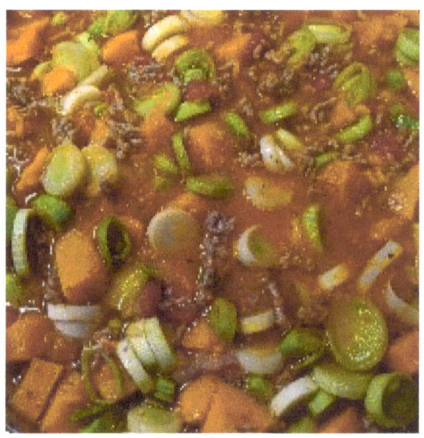

Serving size: 6-8

Ingredients:

- 2 lb hamburger (80-20)
- 2 – 3 carrots
- 1 medium yellow onion
- 2 – 3 potatoes (russet)
- 2 -3 stalks of celery
- 1 can tomato soup with 1 can of water (if you want thinner then add more water)
- 1 can kidney beans, drained

- 1 can black beans, drained
- garlic cloves to taste (we love garlic using 2 - 3 bulbs)
- chili powder to taste * salt and pepper to taste

Directions:

1. Brown hamburger.
2. Add remainder of ingredients.
3. Add chili powder, salt, and pepper to taste.
4. Cook on stove top or in a crock pot depending on your time.
5. If using a crock pot: 2-3 hours on high, or 4-6 hours on low.

✸✸✸

Music: "Hold It Up to the Light" by David Wilcox

"What lies behind us and what lies ahead of us are tiny matters compared to what lives within us."

- Henry David Thoreau

✸✸✸

Day 2 Breakfast

Instant Pot Yogurt Lactose Free

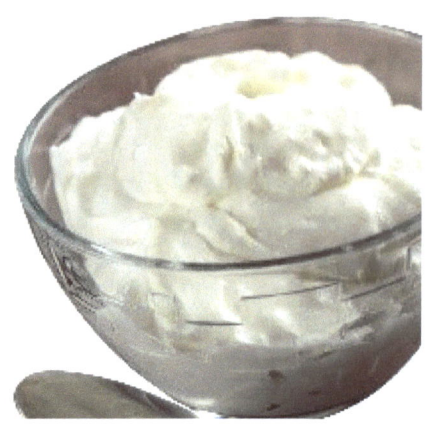

Serving size: 16 - 4 oz. servings

Ingredients:

- 64 oz. container of Fair Life lactose free milk
- 1 can condensed coconut cream for sweetening, if desired (optional if you like your yogurt tarter)
- 1 – 2 tbsp plain yogurt with active culture.

Directions:

1. Add plain yogurt to instant pot, along with condensed milk and lactose free milk. Whisk all together to incorporate yogurt and condensed milk.

2. Select yogurt on the setting panel. Set timer for 10hrs (or 8hrs omitting condensed coconut cream). Close lid making sure vent is closed.

3. When time is up, release vent valve and scoop out yogurt into containers you can refrigerate. I like my yogurt thicker, so I use this Greek yogurt strainer.

4. Place yogurt in this strainer letting whey drain for several days to thicken the yogurt.

***

Music: "Who Better Than Me" (from "Tarzan") by Phil Collins

"Let today be the day you give up who you've been for who you can become."

- Hal Elrod

***

Day 2 Lunch

Tortilla Soup

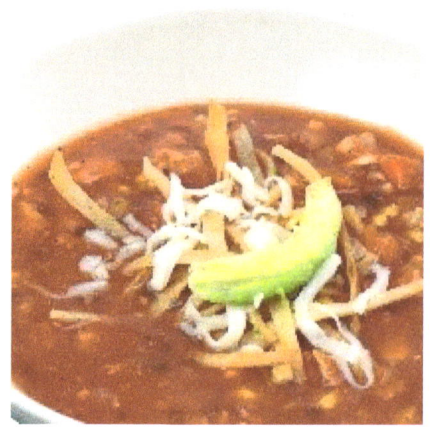

Serving size: 4-6

Ingredients:

- 3 cups (720 ml) chicken broth, heated
- 1 roma tomato or tomato of choice
- 1 carrot, halved
- 1 stalk celery, diced
- 1 onion, sliced
- 1 garlic clove
- 1 yellow squash, sliced
- 1 red bell pepper, sliced

- 1 cabbage, sliced
- 1 mushroom
- 1 tsp taco seasoning
- 1/8 tsp ground cumin
- salt and pepper, to taste

Optional Ingredients:

- 2 oz boneless, skinless chicken breast, cooked, cubed
- ½ jalapeño
- ¼ cup black olives
- ¼ cup frozen or fresh corn
- 2 oz tortilla chips

Garnish Ingredients:

- tortilla chips
- sliced avocado
- shredded mozzarella cheese dairy free

Directions:

1. Place (in this order) broth, tomato, carrot, celery, onion, garlic, squash, pepper, cabbage, mushroom and seasonings into the Vitamix container, secure lid.

2. Turn on Vitamix at Variable 1 speed and slowly increase speed to Variable 10, then to High speed.

3. Blend for 6-7 minutes or until steam escapes from the vented lid.

4. Add optional ingredients (as desired) in this order: chicken, jalapeños, olives, corn, and chips.

5. Turn on at Variable 2 for 1-5 seconds.

6. Remove the lid plug and pour into bowls.

7. Garnish with tortilla chips, avocado, and cheese.

✳✳✳

Music: "Let the Groove Get In" by Justin Timberlake

"We think there is endless time to live but we never know which moment is the last. So share, care, love and celebrate every moment of life."

- Solimar Fiske

✳✳✳

Day 2 Dinner

Keto Beef & Broccoli

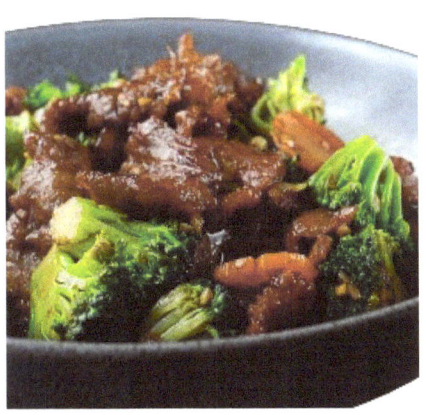

Serving size: 4 Sauce

Ingredients:

- 1 tbsp sesame oil
- 2 garlic cloves minced or minced garlic to taste
- 1 1/4 tsp ground ginger (using a spoon to remove the peel works the best)
- 1 tsp chili paste or 1 teaspoon sweet chili sauce
- 1 pinch red pepper flakes
- 1/2 cup chicken stock or vegetable stock
- 3/4 cup soy sauce

- 1/3 cup honey
- 3 tbsp rice wine vinegar
- 1/3 cup coconut brown sugar packed or regular brown sugar
- 2 tbsp cornstarch
- 2 tbsp water

Main Ingredients:

- olive or avocado oil
- salt and pepper
- 2 steaks trimmed and sliced thin (any type steak or use 1 flank steak)
- 1 head of broccoli (steamed and seasoned with salt and pepper)
- sesame seeds

Directions:

1. In a saucepan over medium heat, add all the sauce ingredients except the cornstarch and water.
2. Heat until boiling.
3. In a small dish, whisk together the cornstarch and water and slowly, while whisking the sauce, pour in the cornstarch water.
4. Continue to whisk and bring back to a boil.
5. Turn down to a simmer and allow to cook for 5-8 minutes.

6. Meanwhile, heat a grill pan or skillet over medium high heat.

7. Season the meat with salt and pepper.

8. Add a drizzle of olive oil onto the hot skillet or pan, and add meat making sure not to crowd the pan.

9. Cook meat for 1-2 minutes, turn over and cook for 1 minute or until almost well done. Note: Overcooking the meat or cooking until well done results in dry chewy meat with less flavor.

10. Place meat on plate and tent with foil while the sauce finishes.

11. Mix beef and sauce together, tossing to coat.

12. Mix beef, sauce and broccoli to the serving bowl.

13. Garnish with sesame seeds.

14. Serve with your choice of rice, noodles or zoodles (best for Keto diet).

We love Panda Express and decided to adapt a much-loved meal! This simple Beef & Broccoli recipe is one of my favorite effortless dinners to make and it all comes together in around 20 minutes!

✳✳✳

Music: "Reach" by Gloria Estefan

"Don't downgrade your dream just to fit your reality. Upgrade your conviction to match your destiny."

- Best Motivational Quotes

✳✳✳

Day 3 Breakfast

Instant Pot Steel Cut Oats

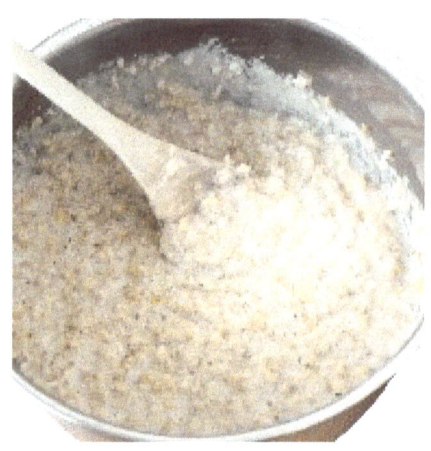

Serving size: 3

Ingredients:

- 3 cups water
- 1 cup steel cut oats — do not use any other kind of oats
- 1/2 teaspoon kosher salt * toppings of choice — fresh fruit, chopped toasted nuts, chia seeds or flaxseeds, maple syrup, agave or honey (or other desired sweetener), splash of almond milk (dairy-free!)

Directions:

1. In a 6-quart Instant Pot, stir together the water, oats, salt.

2. Cover and seal. Cook on HIGH pressure (manual) for 4 minutes.

3. Let the pressure release naturally for 10 minutes. Carefully remove lid.

4. Give the oats a big stir. The oats will continue to thicken as they cool.

5. Ladle into serving bowls and serve hot with any desired toppings.

I've learned some tough news about sweeteners. I try to avoid food or drink that add sucralose, aspartame, Splenda, Nutrasweet or Equal. Gastrointestinal problems and brain damage are real complications to avoid. (Periyasamy, 2019)

✸✸✸

Music: "Also sprach Zarathustra" by Richard Strauss

"At sunrise every soul is born again."

- Muhammad Ali

✸✸✸

Day 3 Lunch

Butternut Squash Soup

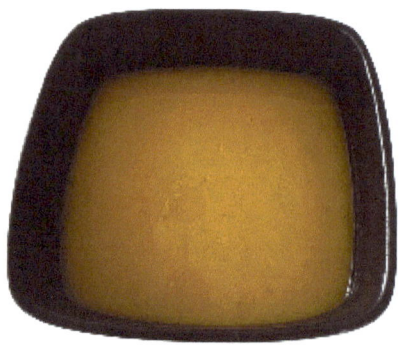

Serving size: 4-6

Ingredients:

- 2 – 3 lb of butternut squash peeled & cubed (the more squash the thicker the soup!)
- 2 tbsp butter
- 1 medium yellow onion
- 6 cups chicken or vegetable broth
- ½ tsp nutmeg or more to taste
- salt and pepper to taste

Directions:

1. Peel and cut up squash into chunks.
2. Use a Dutch oven or heavy stockpot to melt butter.
3. Add onion, cooking until the onion is clear.
4. Add squash and stock.
5. Bring to a boil and reduce to a simmer. Cook for 12–15 minutes or until squash is tender.
6. Remove squash with a slotted spoon and place in a high-speed blender or food processor, adding onions.
7. Blend on high until smooth.
8. Return back to pot and season with nutmeg, salt and pepper.

As you try different types of onions, you will find the soup tastes different. The yellow onion is our preference for our palate.

✳✳✳

Music: "Porscha" by Rippingtons

"Believe that life is worth living and your belief will help create the fact."

- William James

✳✳✳

Day 3 Dinner

Keto Creamy Tuscan Chicken

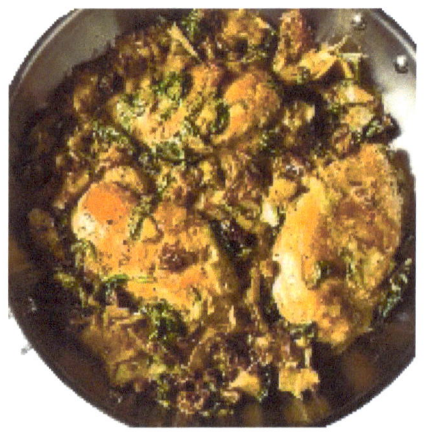

Serving size: 6

Ingredients:

- 1 1/2 lb boneless skinless chicken breasts thinly sliced
- 3 tbsp butter or more if necessary to cook chicken
- 1 cup coconut cream or heavy whipping cream
- 1/2 cup chicken broth
- 8 cloves of garlic, 1.75 oz. or 12 tsps of minced garlic = 4 tbsp
- 1 tsp Italian seasoning
- 1/2 cup goat cheese
- 1 cup spinach, chopped

Directions:

1. Cut chicken into thin slices.
2. Put 2 tbsp butter in a large skillet and cook the chicken on medium heat, 3 -5 minutes per side until chicken is no longer pink.
3. Season w/salt & pepper to taste.
4. Remove chicken to platter and keep warm in the oven.
5. Place 1 tbsp of butter in the pan and add minced garlic. Cook for a minute or until fragrant.
6. Add the coconut cream, chicken broth, Italian seasoning, and goat cheese.
7. Bring to a simmer and whisk over medium heat until it starts to thicken.
8. Add spinach and sun-dried tomatoes.
9. Let simmer until spinach starts to wilt.
10. Add chicken back in and cover with sauce.
11. Serve over zucchini noodles (best for Keto diet aka "zoodles" which are sauteed after zucchini is prepared using the vegetable spiralizer), spaghetti squash (baked and scooped out) or choice of rice.

✳✳✳

Music: "Clair de Lune" by Claude Debussy

"Shoot for the moon. Even if you miss, you'll land among the stars."

- Les Brown

✳✳✳

Day 4 Breakfast

Eggs Benedict with Hollandaise Sauce Gluten & Dairy Free

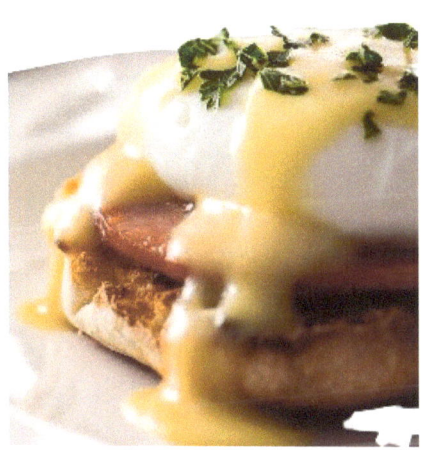

Serving size: 4 Sauce

Ingredients:

- 3 eggs yolks
- 1 tbsp Lemon juice
- 1/2 tsp salt
- 1/8 tsp cayenne pepper (optional)
- 10 tbsp unsalted butter Main Ingredients:
- 1 pkg. english muffin gluten free, cut in half

- 1 pkg. canadian bacon
- distilled white vinegar
- paprika
- parsley

Sauce Directions:

1. Melt the butter on the stove top or microwave making sure not to boil as to retain the moisture.
2. Add the egg yolks, lemon juice, salt & cayenne into a blender.
3. Blend on medium high speed until egg yolks lighten in color.
4. Once lightened turn blender speed to lowest setting and slowly add the melted butter.
5. Continue blending until all materials are incorporated. Makes approximately 1 cup sauce.
6. Keep warm until ready to use or it will solidify.
7. Remainder can be stored in the refrigerator and used as a spread for up to a week.

Main Dish Directions:

1. Cook Canadian bacon in a fry pan until heated through.
2. Cover and set aside.
3. Toast the English muffins while you're cooking the bacon, setting on plates or a serving platter.

4. Crack open the number of eggs you desire and put in individual ramekins.

5. In a large frying pan add 2-3 inches of water with 4 – 5 teaspoons of the vinegar.

6. Bring to a boil and gently add eggs to boiling water.

7. Cook 3 – 5 minutes not overcrowding the pan.

8. While eggs are cooking, begin assembly.

9. Place one slice of Canadian bacon on each toasted English muffin.

10. Gently remove each poached egg from the pan with a slotted spoon and place directly on Canadian bacon from water when done to desired consistency.

11. Pour hollandaise sauce over poached egg and (optional) sprinkle with paprika and parsley.

12. Repeat the process until all are assembled - and enjoy!

This is by far Judith's most preferred breakfast. Once you get used to the assembly line requirement, you can easily serve this often!

✳✳✳

Music: "Here Comes the Sun" by The Beatles

"The sun is a daily reminder that we too can rise again from the darkness. That we too can shine our own light."

- Sara Aina

***

Day 4 Lunch

Keto Lettuce Wraps

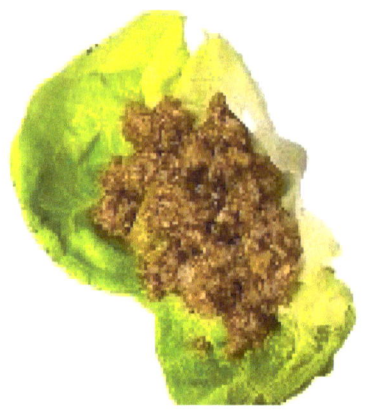

Serving size: 8

Ingredients:

- 1 lb ground turkey

- 1 tbsp avocado oil

- 1 tbsp sesame oil

- 1 large yellow onion diced small

- 1/3 cup hoisin sauce

- 2 tbsp soy sauce

- 1 tbsp rice wine vinegar
- 1 tbsp Asian chili garlic sauce
- 3 cloves of garlic minced or (3 tbsp minced garlic)
- 1 tsp ground ginger powder or 2 tsp freshly grated ginger
- 1 – 8 oz can water chestnuts drained and minced (I mince mine in a blender with enough water covering the water chestnut then drain them)
- 2 – 3 green onions, cut fine
- ½ tsp salt or more to taste
- ½ tsp pepper or more to taste
- 1 head of butter lettuce

Directions:

1. In a large wok or skillet add oils and turkey.
2. Cook over medium high heat until turkey is cooked through.
3. Add onion, hoisin sauce, soy sauce, rice wine vinegar, and chili garlic sauce.
4. Stir to combine and cook for 4-5 minutes until onion is soft and translucent, and most of the liquid is absorbed.
5. Add garlic and ginger, stirring to combine and cook for several more minutes.

6. Add water chestnuts, green onions, salt, and pepper.

7. Cook for additional 1-2 minutes.

8. Spoon mixture into the lettuce leaves and serve.

I adapted PF Chang's recipe for lettuce wraps so we could eat this delicious, light meal anytime we desire!

✼✼✼

Music: "Shake It Out" by Florence & the Machine

"One of the purposes of life is to let go of all that baggage you're dragging around and be free again."

- Neil Strauss

✼✼✼

Day 4 Dinner

Keto Instant Pot Ribs

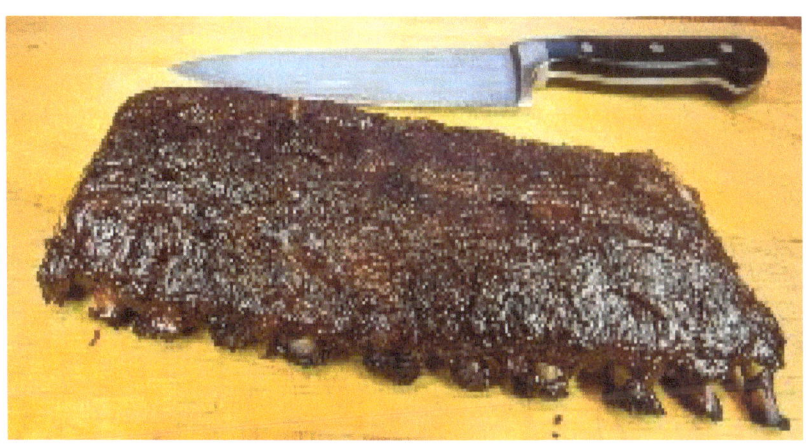

Serving size: 4

Ingredients:

- 3 lb baby back ribs or pork loin ribs
- 6 cups apple juice
- ¼ cup apple cider vinegar
- ½ tsp liquid smoke optional
- 1 tbsp seasoning salt
- 2 tbsp BBQ dry rub

- 2/3 cup sweet BBQ sauce, divided

Directions:

1. Pat dry the rack of ribs with a paper towel and rub dry ingredients on both sides.

2. In the Instant Pot, combine apple juice, vinegar, liquid smoke and 1/3 cup of BBQ sauce.

3. Coil the rack of ribs inside the Instant Pot with the bone-side facing the center. Ribs should all be partially submerged.

4. Cook on high pressure for 25 minutes, followed by a 10 minute natural pressure release before manually releasing remaining pressure.

5. Using two sets of tongs, carefully transfer ribs to a rimmed baking sheet lined with a wire rack, with the meat side up.

6. Brush the top and sides with the remaining 1/3 cup BBQ sauce.

7. Broil in the center of the oven on high for 4-5 minutes.

8. Remove from the oven and let rest for 5-10 min before serving.

9. Serve with more BBQ sauce if desired.

Instant Pot Ribs is the easiest way to achieve tender, juicy ribs.

Whether you're using baby back ribs, pressure cooking tenderizes the meat in a fraction of the time.

✳✳✳

Music: "Cello Suite No.1 in G Major: ll. Allemande" by Johann S. Bach

"For to be free is not merely to cast off one's chains, but to live in a way that respects and enhances the freedom of others."

- Nelson Mandela

✳✳✳

Day 5 Breakfast

Vegan Mango Kale Smoothie with Banana Nut Bread Gluten & Dairy Free

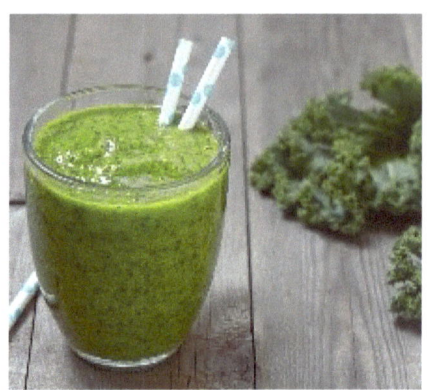

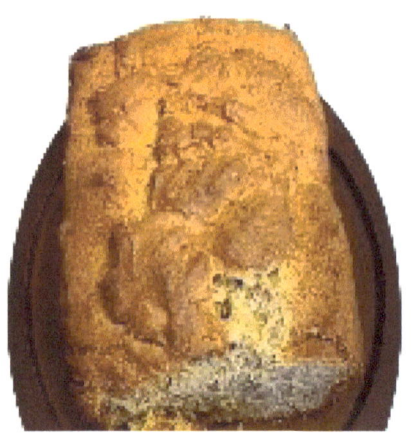

Serving size: 1 – 18 oz (smoothie), 16 slices (bread)

Smoothie Ingredients:

- 1 Banana
- 1/2 cup mango juice (Naked Mighty Mango brand is best!)
- 1/4 cup apple juice
- 1/3 cup frozen kale
- 1/8 cup chopped almonds or almond flour, or 1 tbsp almond butter
- 1 scoop vegan protein powder of choice (dairy & gluten free)
- Ice

Smoothie Directions:

1. Add as much ice as you would like. The more ice the thicker and colder the smoothie will be.
2. Add in this order: banana, mango juice, apple juice, kale, almonds and protein powder.
3. Blend and enjoy this vegan mango kale recipe!

Bread Ingredients:

- ½ cup butter
- ¾ cup sugar
- 2 eggs
- 1 tsp vanilla

- 3 bananas, large, mashed
- 2 cups rice flour
- ¼ cup vegan protein powder
- 2 tsp baking powder
- ½ cup pecans, chopped, (I pulse in blender for several seconds)

Bread Directions:

1. Preheat oven to 325°F.
2. In a large bowl, cream butter and sugar.
3. Beat in eggs, vanilla and bananas.
4. Stir in flour, protein powder and baking powder until moistened.
5. Stir in pecans.
6. Pour into a greased 5 × 9 inch loaf pan.
7. Bake for 1 hour and 20 minutes.
8. Let cool 10 minutes before removing from pan, then slice and serve.

Smoothie King started a new line of taste treats with this one a winner for us - adapted to drink anytime desired, and especially after working out!

✳✳✳

Music: "Thank You for This Day" by Karen Drucker

"Welcome each day with gratitude and joy."

– Pinterest

✳✳✳

Day 5 Lunch

Chili with Cornbread Egg, Gluten & Dairy Free

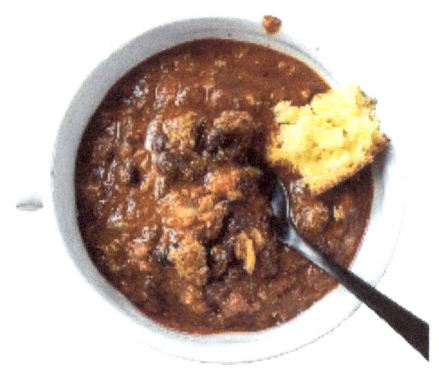

Serving size: 8-10

Chili Ingredients:

- 1 lb ground beef or turkey
- 1 lb ground sausage or turkey sausage
- 1 28 oz can diced tomatoes
- 2 cans chili beans with sauce
- 2 cans kidney beans drained
- 2 cans black beans drained
- 1 - 7 oz can diced green chiles (optional)

- 1 medium onion (we prefer yellow), diced fine
- 2 cans 10.5 oz tomato soup
- chili powder to taste
- worcestershire sauce
- garlic powder

Cornbread Ingredients:

- 1 cup yellow cornmeal
- 1-1/2 cups rice flour
- 3 tsp baking powder
- 1 tsp salt
- 3 tbs sugar add little more if you want more sweetness
- 1/2 cup butter melted
- 6 tbsp applesauce or lactose free yogurt
- 1 cup almond milk dairy free
- 1 tsp vanilla extract

Chili Directions:

1. Brown hamburger and sausage in a 7 qt cast iron pot.
2. Season with salt, pepper, garlic powder, chile powder and worcestershire sauce.
3. Add onion and cook until most of the juice is incorporated into

the meat.

4. Drain any excess fat off.

5. Add tomatoes, chili beans, kindey beans, green chiles and tomato soup.

6. Season with more chili powder to taste.

7. Mix all together and add 1 can of water. If you like your chili thinner add more water, or thicker add less water.

8. Bring to a boil, then reduce to a simmer and cook for 30-45 minutes.

9. Taste and add additional salt, pepper and chili powder to taste.

Cornbread Directions:

1. Preheat the oven to 350 degrees.

2. In a large bowl, mix together all dry ingredients - cornmeal, flour, salt, baking powder and sugar.

3. In another bowl, add the melted butter and applesauce (or yogurt), milk and vanilla extract and mix everything together until well combined.

4. Add the butter mixture to the dry flour mixture and mix the contents together without forming any lumps. In case the batter is too thick (as it may depend on the cornmeal and flour you use), you may add a little more milk and mix again(just add one tablespoon of extra milk at a time and then mix and see if you need more). You can use a balloon whisk to mix the ingredients to blend in perfectly.

5. Grease oil or melted butter in a square pan and pour the cornbread batter into it.

6. Bake the cornbread for 25 to 30 minutes until the top is lightly browned and the inside is cooked.

7. Check cornbread by inserting a toothpick at the center of the cornbread which should come out clean. If the inside is not cooked enough, cover the pan with foil and cook for a few more minutes until the cornbread is cooked completely. Cover with the foil to prevent the cornbread from drying out.

8. Allow the bread to cool down, then cut and serve the warm cornbread with honey butter - or jam or syrup as desired.

We certainly have differences of spicy hot preferences. I love spice – the more the better. Judith does not like spicy hot at all. So the jalapeño is not found in my chili! Judith absolutely loves Marie Callendar's cornbread, but cannot eat it as it's not gluten free. So I found this super yummy recipe. If you truly have a dairy allergy, you will want to use applesauce instead of lactose free yogurt as it's still milk, just no lactase enzyme required to break it down in the gut.

✳✳✳

Music: "Butterflies and Hurricanes" by Muse

"The pessimist complains about the wind; the optimist expects it to change; the realist adjusts the sails."

- William Arthur Ward

✳✳✳

Day 5 Dinner

Instant Pot Dal

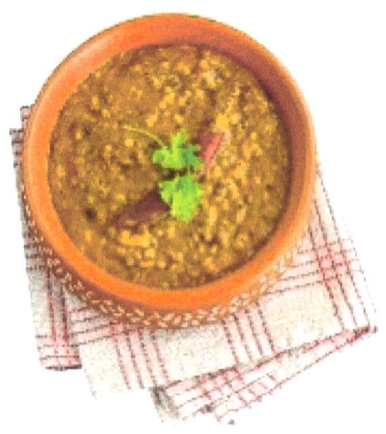

Serving size: 4

Ingredients:

- 1 large yellow onion diced
- 2 tbsp coconut oil
- 1 tbsp ginger minced
- 4 cloves of garlic minced or 2 large tbsp minced garlic
- 1 tsp cumin
- 1 tsp turmeric
- 1 tbsp yellow curry powder
- 1 tsp garam marsala

- ¼ tsp cayenne or more for more heat
- ¼ tsp mustard seeds
- 1 ½ cups red lentils
- 3 cups water
- ½ tsp salt
- 2 medium tomatoes chopped
- ¼ cup fresh cilantro chopped with some extra for garnish
- 1 jalepeno pepper (optional)

Directions:

1. On the instant pot select sauté, add oil, when hot add onion and cook until clear.
2. Stir in garlic, cumin, turmeric, curry powder, garam marsala, cayenne, and mustard seeds. Cook until fragrant.
3. Hit cancel, then add lentils, water, salt, and chopped tomatoes. Mix well.
4. Close instant pot lid make sure release valve is closed. Select pressure cook on high for 10 minutes.
5. Wait 10 more minutes for pot to release then you can open valve to manually release the balance of steam.
6. Stir lentil mixture and add cilantro.
7. Serve over any type of rice and garnish with cilantro and jalepeno pepper (optional).

Masoor Dal used to be one of the meals Judith loved to cook, and then I found this new, quicker, easy, more tasty recipe we both love to eat!

✸✸✸

Music: "Unwritten" by Natasha Bedingfield

"Can you remember who you were before the world told you who you should be?"

- Unknown

✸✸✸

Day 6 Breakfast

Biscuits and Gravy Gluten & Dairy Free

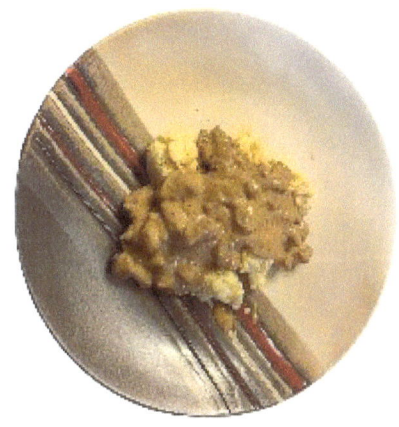

Serving size: 4

Biscuits Ingredients:

- 2 cups rice flour
- 2 tsp baking powder
- ½ tsp baking soda
- ½ tsp salt
- ¼ cup shortening
- ¾ cup almond milk

Gravy Ingredients:

- 1 lb package pork sausage or sausage of choice, turkey, chicken
- 2 tbsp butter
- 2-3 tbsp rice flour
- 1/8 tsp sea salt
- 1 ¼ - 1 1/3 cups almond milk

Biscuit Directions:

1. In a bowl, combine the flour, baking powder, baking soda and salt.
2. Cut in shortening until the mixture resembles coarse crumbs.
3. Stir in milk and mix together until a ball is formed. If it is too dry or not coming together add a dash more milk.
4. Spoon out onto a greased baking sheet.
5. Bake at 450° for 10 – 15 minutes or until golden brown.

Gravy Directions:

- In a large skillet, cook sausage over medium heat until no longer pink.
- Drain excess grease.
- Add butter and heat until melted.
- Add flour, salt, and pepper.

- Cook and stir until well blended.
- Gradually add in the milk, stirring constantly.
- Bring to a boil and cook until thickened.
- Serve over the biscuits.

This egg-free recipe is favored especially by Judith's dad Frank because he loves biscuits and gravy and is highly allergic to eggs. When I cook this for him he insists on taking extra helpings home!

❋❋❋

Music: "Live Like You Were Dying" (from "The Bucket List") by Tim McGraw

"Every day is an opportunity to make a new happy ending."

- Author Unknown

❋❋❋

Day 6 Lunch

Keto Zucchini Ravioli Dairy Free

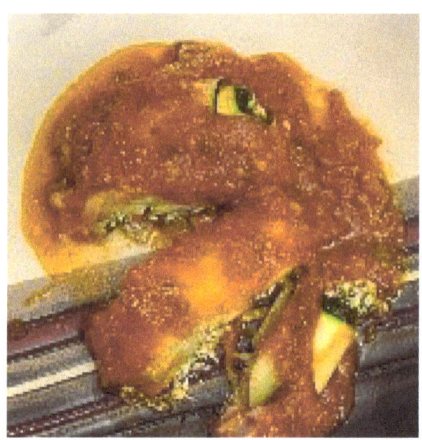

Serving size: 6

Ingredients:

- 2 medium zucchinis
- olive oil to taste
- 2 cloves garlic minced or 2 1/2 - 3 tsp
- 2 cups chopped fresh spinach
- 1 cup goat cheese (or ricotta cheese if you don't need it dairy free)
- 2 tbsp fresh basil
- salt to taste

- pepper to taste
- 1 cup marinara sauce
- 1/2 cup shredded mozzarella goat cheese (or just mozarella cheese if you don't need it dairy free)

Directions:

1. Preheat oven to 425°.
2. Cut ends of zucchini, then use a mandolin to slice zucchini into wide strips with desired thickness.
3. Put zucchini strips onto a separate plate and layer 2 strips vertically & 2 strips horizontally to make a cross.
4. Heat pan over medium-high heat. Add olive oil then garlic and sauté until fragrant, about a minute.
5. Add spinach, salt & pepper.
6. Sauté until spinach is wilted, 1 - 2 minutes.
7. Remove from heat & allow to cool for 10 minutes.
8. In a large bowl add spinach & garlic. Then add cheese, basil, salt & pepper. Mix well until combined.
9. Using a spoon, scoop about 1 tbsp of mixture and place in the middle of each zucchini noodle cross. (I found the size of the zucchini ravioli will be determined by the amount of mixture you scoop into the cross.)

10. Fold each side of the cross to seal mixture & flip so seam side is down.

11. In a baking dish pour the marinara sauce & smooth out.

12. Place evenly the zucchini raviolis then top with more cheese.

13. Bake 15 - 20 minutes.

14. Sprinkle fresh basil over top after removing from the oven.

This nutritious meal replaces Judith's craving for Chef Boyardee's processed gluten ravioli - and she loves this so much better!

✳✳✳

Music: "Riverdance" (Dance Reprise) by Bill Whelan

"Steps are only steps unless you are brave enough to open up your soul and become one with the music, the story and the people around you."

- Katrina Meske

✳✳✳

Day 6 Dinner:

Pasta e Fagioli Soup Gluten Free

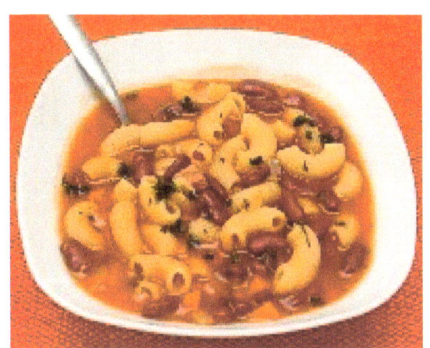

Serving size: 6

Ingredients:

- 1 lb ground beef
- 1 small onions, chopped
- 1 large carrots, slivered
- 3 stalks celery, diced
- 2 cloves garlic, minced
- 2 14.5 oz can diced tomatoes
- 1 15 oz can red kidney beans w/liquid

- 1 15oz can great northern beans w/liquid
- 1 12 oz can tomato sauce
- 1 12 oz can V-8 juice
- 1 tbsp white vinegar
- ½ tsp dried oregano
- 1 tsp dried basil
- ½ teaspoons pepper
- ½ tsp dried thyme
- ½ lb ditalini pasta or gluten free pasta

Directions:

1. Brown the ground beef in a large saucepan over medium heat. Drain off the excess fat.
2. Add onion, carrot, celery and garlic, sauté for 10 minutes.
3. Add remaining ingredients except the pasta and simmer for 1 hour.
4. After 50 minutes into the process cook the pasta according to the directions until al dente. Drain but don't rinse.
5. Add the pasta to the pot and simmer for an additional 5 – 10 minutes.
6. Ready to serve.

This recipe has been modified and refined from our restaurant experience at Olive Garden. Truly tastes like the restaurant experience - avoid making any slow cooker version!

✳︎✳︎✳︎

Music: "Dream" by Priscilla Ahn

"Cherish your yesterdays, dream your tomorrows and live your todays."

- Anonymous

✳︎✳︎✳︎

Day 7 Breakfast

Overnight French Toast Gluten Free

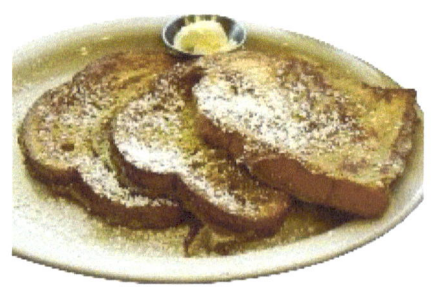

Serving size: 6-8

Ingredients:

- ¼ cup melted butter (4 tbsps)
- ¾ cup coconut brown sugar
- 1 loaf bread gluten free
- 8 eggs slightly beaten
- 1 cup almond milk
- 1 tbsp vanilla extract
- 1 tsp cinnamon
- ¼ tsp ginger powder

- 1/8 tsp nutmeg
- 1/8 tsp sea salt
- ½ cup pecans chopped (chop in a blender to desired consistency)
- syrup (optional)
- powdered sugar (optional)

Directions:

1. In a bowl combine melted butter and brown sugar.
2. Mix until brown sugar is totally coated, then pour into a 9x 13 baking dish.
3. Arrange bread in the baking dish, overlapping is okay to get more bread in.
4. Combine milk, eggs, vanilla, cinnamon, ginger, nutmeg, and salt.
5. Blend well and pour over, making sure to get all the bread covered.
6. Cover with plastic wrap and refrigerate 4-12 hours. It is better if it can sit overnight.
7. In the morning take out of the refrigerator and let stand on the counter while preheating the oven to 350°.
8. Bake for 30-35 minutes checking to see the top is not getting too dark. Use foil if necessary, to reduce the darkness.
9. Remove from oven and sprinkle with powdered sugar if desired. I find syrup is not needed but can be used if desired.

Judith loves the bread texture of the Franz 7-grain gluten free brand. I make half a pan with her bread and half a pan with my gluten bread. Our dear friend LaQuel invited us for Christmas breakfast one year and was so sure of her culinary skill that she didn't even ask what we liked! She was sooo right on! This recipe was shared by her – thank you, LaQuel!

❋❋❋

Music: "Best Day of My Life" by American Authors

"The sun will rise and set regardless. What we choose to do with the light while it's here is up to us."

- Alexandra Elle

❋❋❋

Day 7 Lunch

Fish Sticks

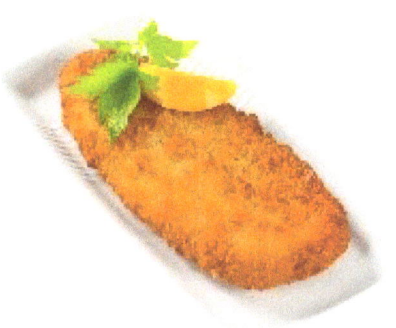

Serving size: 4

Ingredients:

- 1/2 cup crushed pork rinds
- 1/2 tsp salt
- 1/2 tsp paprika
- 1/2 tsp lemon pepper
- 1/2 cup coconut flour
- 1 large egg, beaten
- 3/4 lb cod fillets, cut down the middle

- cooking spray or oil
- parsley garnish
- lemon garnish

Directions:

1. Preheat oven to 400°.
2. In a bowl, mix pork rinds & seasonings.
3. Place flour & egg in separate bowls.
4. Dip fish in flour to coat both sides, shake off excess.
5. Dip in egg wash, then in pork rinds until fully coated.
6. Place on a foil lined baking sheet that has been sprayed or oiled.
7. Bake for 10 - 12 minutes then check. If more time is needed, turn and bake several more minutes.
8. Once fish begins to flake, fish sticks are done.
9. Garnish each fish stick with parsely and sliced lemon.

✳✳✳

Music: "What a Feeling" from "Flashdance" by Irene Cara

"If you can't figure out your purpose, figure out your passion. For your passion will lead you right into your purpose."

- Bishop T. D. Jakes

✳✳✳

Day 7 Dinner

Keto Asian Cabbage Stir Fry

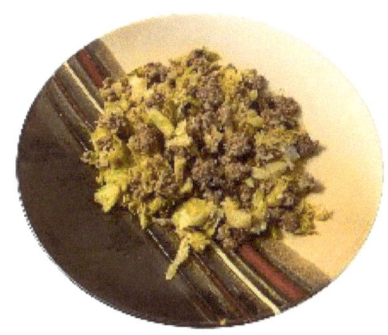

Serving size: 6-8

Ingredients:

- 25 oz green cabbage
- 8 oz butter
- 25 oz ground beef 80/20 (or other ground meat of choice)
- 1 tsp onion powder
- 1 tsp salt
- ¼ tsp black pepper (or white pepper to make it spicier)
- 1 tbsp white wine vinegar or white vinegar

- 2 garlic cloves or 1 heaping tbsp, or more depending on your love of garlic

- 3 green onions or scallions if available, diced

- 1 tsp chili flakes (more or less depending on your desired level of spicy heat)

- 1 tbsp fresh ginger, minced

- 1 tbsp sesame oil

Directions:

1. Shred cabbage in food processor or with a knife.

2. Fry the cabbage in 5 oz. of butter in a large skillet or wok on medium high heat. Make sure not to burn the cabbage. Cabbage is done when it softens.

3. Add spices and vinegar to cabbage, mixing well.

4. Place cabbage in a large bowl.

5. Use the cabbage skillet or use another pan to melt the remaining 3 oz of butter.

6. Add garlic, chili flakes and ginger, sautéing for several minutes.

7. Add ground meat and brown until thoroughly cooked through and most of the juices have evaporated.

8. Lower the heat and mix in green onions and cabbage until hot. If needed add more salt and pepper to taste.

9. Top with sesame oil and serve.

When we decided to try a Keto diet, this meal was a staple which we continue to love and sometimes add a bed of rice underneath it.

✳✳✳

Music: "Leyenda" by Andres Segovia

"Legends are not born. Being a legend is all about living life like a legend."

- Nishant Jain

✳✳✳

Chapter 10

21 Music & Quotes for Relaxation & Positive Mindset

Dennis has inspired me to consider how stress impacts gut health. Here are some music listening suggestions to deepen relaxation and keep a positive mindset - not just any music will do. The Music 4 Life® Music Medicine Protocol is considered an alternative therapy which I developed over the past decades.

As a board-certified music therapist, I've learned so much working with more than 11,000 patients in residential addiction treatment centers, documenting over 35,000 experiences. They've taught me about the impact toxic music can have on mental health (anxiety and depression) as well as lifespan development. I discovered what they could do about it, guided by their insights.

Utilizing the Music Medicine Protocol can keep you centered, as well as physically and emotionally flexible, with an ever present optimistic mental attitude. This translates into developing emotional fluidity - 99% of the time - staying emotionally and mentally flexible and optimistic, no matter what! You will find life-affirming quotes and motivating music at the end of each designated recipe. Designed for both men and women, the following tip focuses on how to reduce anxiety and depression.

With or without lyric, twenty-one music selections that follow are noted as validating unsettled feelings, then shifting to soothing or energizing moods. This may help heal feelings of anxiety or depression, or shift you into a more energized, positive mindset, thereby reducing the intensity of unsettledness. Consider listening more than one time to each selection for maximum impact.

If you find that anxiety or depression is not managed with this music (and after several consecutive listening's), I recommend you take advantage of this book's Special Offer to learn how music may be toxic and what to do about it. And, consult with your mental health professional to avoid injurious behaviors. - Judith Pinkerton

7 BREAKFAST MUSIC & QUOTES

Day 1 "Psyche" by Chris Spheeris to support a soothing, mildly energizing positive mood.

"We can only appreciate the miracle of a sunrise if we have waited in the darkness."

- Sapra Reddy

Day 2 "Who Better Than Me" (from "Tarzan") by Phil Collins to support an energized positive mood.

"Let today be the day you give up who you've been for who you can become."

- Hal Elrod

Day 3 "Also sprach Zarathustra" by Richard Strauss to validate unsettled feelings, then shift into supporting a soothing, mildly energizing positive mood.

"At sunrise every soul is born again."

- Muhammad Ali

Day 4 "Here Comes the Sun" by The Beatles to support an energized positive mood.

"The sun is a daily reminder that we too can rise again from the darkness. That we too can shine our own light."

- Sara Aina

Day 5 "Thank You for This Day" by Karen Drucker to support a soothing, mildly energizing positive mood.

"Welcome each day with gratitude and joy."

– Pinterest

Day 6 "Live Like You Were Dying" (from "The Bucket List") by Tim McGraw to support a soothing, mildly energizing positive mood.

"Every day is an opportunity to make a new happy ending."

- Author Unknown

Day 7 "Best Day of My Life" by American Authors to support an energizing positive mood.

"The sun will rise and set regardless. What we choose to do with the light while it's here is up to us."

- Alexandra Elle

7 LUNCHES MUSIC & QUOTES

Day 1 "Feeling Good" by Michael Bubleto support a soothing, mildly energizing positive mood.

"As you think thoughts that feel good to you, you will be in harmony with who you really are."

- Abraham Hicks

Day 2 "Let the Groove Get In" by Justin Timberlake to support an energized positive mood.

"We think there is endless time to live but we never know which moment is the last. So share, care, love and celebrate every moment of life."

- Solimar Fiske

Day 3 "Porscha" by Rippingtons to support an energized positive mood.

"Believe that life is worth living and your belief will help create the fact."

- William James

Day 4 "Shake It Out" by Florence & the Machine to validate unsettled feelings, then shift into supporting a soothing, mildly energizing positive mood.

"One of the purposes of life is to let go of all that baggage you're dragging around and be free again."

- Neil Strauss

Day 5 "Butterflies and Hurricanes" by Muse to validate unsettled feelings, then shift into supporting a soothing, mildly energizing positive mood.

"The pessimist complains about the wind; the optimist expects it to change; the realist adjusts the sails."

- William Arthur Ward

Day 6 "Riverdance" (Dance Reprise) by Bill Whelan to support an energized positive mood.

"Steps are only steps unless you are brave enough to open up your soul and become one with the music, the story and the people around you."

- Katrina Meske

Day 7 "What a Feeling" from "Flashdance" by Irene Cara to validate any unsettled feelings of depression, then support a shift into soothing feelings, then an energized positive mood.

"If you can't figure out your purpose, figure out your passion. For your passion will lead you right into your purpose."

- Bishop T. D. Jakes

✽✽✽

7 DINNERS MUSIC & QUOTES

Day 1 "Hold It Up to the Light" by David Wilcoxto support a soothing mood.

"What lies behind us and what lies ahead of us are tiny matters compared to what lives within us."

- Henry David Thoreau

Day 2 "Reach" by Gloria Estefan to support a soothing, mildly energizing positive mood.

"Don't downgrade your dream just to fit your reality. Upgrade your conviction to match your destiny."

- Best Motivational Quotes

Day 3 "Clair de Lune" by Claude Debussy to support a soothing mood.

"Shoot for the moon. Even if you miss, you'll land among the stars."

- Les Brown

Day 4 "Cello Suite No.1 in G Major: ll. Allemande" by Johann S. Bach to support a soothing mood.

"For to be free is not merely to cast off one's chains, but to live in a way that respects and enhances the freedom of others."

- Nelson Mandela

Day 5 "Unwritten" by Natasha Bedingfieldto support an energized positive mood.

"Can you remember who you were before the world told you who you should be?"

- Unknown

Day 6 "Dream" by Priscilla Ahn to support a soothing, mildly energizing positive mood.

"Cherish your yesterdays, dream your tomorrows and live your todays."

- Anonymous

Day 7 "Leyenda" by Andres Segovia to support an energized mood.

"Legends are not born. Being a legend is all about living life like a legend."

- Nishant Jain

Special Offer

When you want to learn more about reducing anxiety and depression, take this eCourse to learn how to decode whether your music is toxic or not. Find tips about healthy or hungry music listening habits that teeter on danger zones, with evidence based on psychology, neuroscience and music therapy.

At MusicMedicineAcademy.com a holistic approach deals with lifespan development in the eCourses. Enroll in "Is Your Music Toxic?" and get free access with this coupon code: TOXICMUSICNOTMEE.

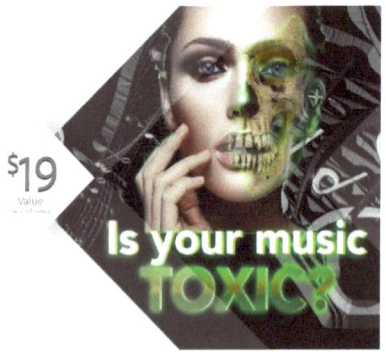

References

5 ways to boost your immune system through your gut. (n.d.). DuPage Medical Group. Retrieved from https://www.dupagemedicalgroup.com/health-topic/5-ways-to-boost-your-immune-system-through-your-gut

Alkasir, R., Li, J., Li, X., Jin, M., & Zhu, B. (2017). Human gut microbiota: the links with dementia development. Protein & cell, 8(2), 90–102. https://doi.org/10.1007/s13238-016-0338-6

American Psychological Association. (2018, November 1). Stress effects on the body. Retrieved from http://www.apa.org/topics/stress/body

Ariciu, G. (n.d.). Leaky gut, inflammation and anxiety. Ozark Holistic Center. Retrieved on December 13, 2020 from https://ozarkholisticcenter.com/blog/leaky-gut-inflammation-and-anxiety/

Arthritis by the numbers. (2019). Arthritis Foundation, 3, 4100.17.10445. https://www.arthritis.org/gemedia/e1256607-fa87-4593-aa8a-8db4f291072a/2019-abtn-final-march-2019.pdf

Bittman, B. B., Berk, L. S., Felten, D. L., Westengard, J., Simonton, O. C., Pappas, J., & Ninehouser, M. (2001). Composite effects of group drumming music therapy on modulation of neuroendocrine-immune parameters in normal subjects. Alternative therapies in health and medicine, 7(1), 38–47.

Bittman, B., Bruhn, K. T., Stevens, C., Westengard, J., & Umbach, P. O. (2003). Recreational music-making: a cost-effective group interdisciplinary strategy for reducing burnout and improving mood states in long-term care workers. Advances in mind-body medicine, 19(3-4), 4–15.

Can gut bacteria improve your health? (October, 2016). Harvard Health Publishing. Retrieved from https://www.health.harvard.edu/staying-healthy/can-gut-bacteria-improve-your-health

Carvalho, F.R., Wang, Q., van Ee, R., Persoone, D., & Spence, C. (2017). Music modulates the perceived creaminess, sweetness, and bitterness of chocolate. Appetite, 108, 383-390. https://doi.org/10.1016/j.appet.2016.10.026

Chaput, J.P., Klingenberg, L., Astrup, A. & Sjödin, A.M. (2011). Modern sedentary activities promote overconsumption of food in our current obesogenic environment. Obesity Reviews, 12: e12-e20. https://doi.org/10.1111/j.1467-789X.2010.00772.x

Clapp, M., Aurora, N., Herrera, L., Bhatia, M., Wilen, E., & Wakefield, S. (2017). Gut microbiota's effect on mental health: The gut-brain axis. Clinics and Practice, 7(4). https://doi.org/10.4081/cp.2017.987

Dix, M. (2020, August 20). What's an unhealthy gut? How gut health affects you. Healthline. Retrieved from https://www.healthline.com/health/gut-health#signs-and-symptoms

Fraser, C. (2018, March 7). 10 signs you have leaky gut syndrome and how to heal it naturally. LiveLoveFruit. Retrieved from https://livelovefruit.com/10-signs-leaky-gut-syndrome/#:~:text=%20How%20To%20Repair%20Leaky%20Gut%20Syndrome%20and,foods.%20 2%20Reduce%20Your%20Stress%20Load%20More%20

Gundry, S. (2018, May 25). Diet expert reveals all: It's like a powerwash for your insides! Gundrey MD. Retrieved from https://thenewgutfix.com/191227A.php?src=bing

Gupta, R.S., Warren, C.M., Smith, B.M., Jiang, J., Blumenstock, J.A., Davis, M.M., Schleimer, R.P. & Nadeau, K.C. (2019, January 4). Prevalence and severity of food allergies among US adults. JAMA Netw Open, 2(1), doi:10.1001/jamanetworkopen.2018.5630. Retrieved from https://jamanetwork.com/journals/jamanetworkopen/fullarticle/2720064

Hitti, M. (2004, December 23). A healthy gut may resist allergies, asthma. WebMD. Retrieved from https://www.webmd.com/allergies/news/20041223/healthy-gut-may-resist-allergies-asthma

Lin, Y.H.T.;, Hamid, N., Shepherd, D., Kantono, K., & Spence, C. (2019). Environmental sounds influence the multisensory perception of chocolate gelati. Foods, 8, 124. https://doi.org/10.3390/foods8040124

McMillen, M. (n.d.). Leaky gut syndrome: What is it? WebMD. Retrieved on December 13, 2020 from https://www.webmd.com/digestive-disorders/features/leaky-gut-syndrome#1

Stone, S. (2020, March 23). Does gut health really affect skin health? The Aedition. Retrieved from https://aedit.com/aedition/relationship-between-unhealthy-gut-microbiome-skin-conditions

Periyasamy, A. (2019, January). Artificial sweeteners. International Journal of Research and Review, 6(1). Retrieved from https://www.ijrrjournal.com/IJRR_Vol.6_Issue.1_Jan2019/IJRR0019.pdf

Stroebele, N. & de Castro, J.M. (2006, November). Listening to music while eating is related to increases in people's food intake and meal duration. Appetite, 47(3), 285-289. https://doi.org/10.1016/j.

appet.2006.04.001

Torgan, C. (2013, November 25). Gut microbes linked to rheumatoid arthritis. NIH Research Matters. Retrieved from https://www.nih.gov/news-events/nih-research-matters/gut-microbes-linked-rheumatoid-arthritis

Underwood, E. (September 20, 2018). Your gut is directly connected to your brain, by a newly discovered neuron circuit. American Association for the Advancement of Science. Retrieved from https://www.sciencemag.org/news/ 2018/09/your-gut-directly-connected-your-brain-newly-discovered-neuron-circuit

University of Zurich. (2018, October 11). Link between gut flora and multiple sclerosis discovered. ScienceDaily. Retrieved from www.sciencedaily.com/releases/2018/10/181011103636.htm

Zhang, Y., Li, S., Gan, R., Zhou, T., Xu, D., & Li, H. (2015, April). Impacts of gut bacteria on human health and diseases. International Journal of Molecular Sciences, 16(4), 7493–7519. https://doi.org/10.3390/ijms16047493

About The Authors

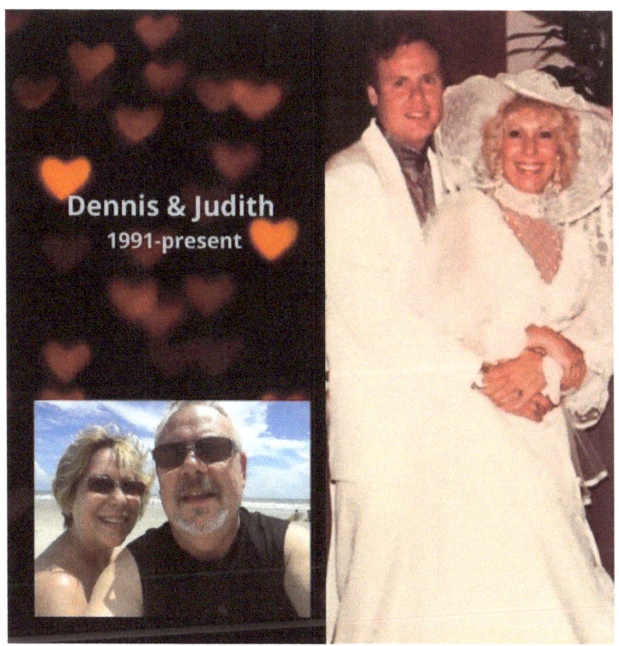

Dennis D. Burkhardt & Judith Pinkerton

celebrating 30 years marriage in 2021!

Dennis is a retired chiropractor, nutrition specialist, sports official, educator and life-long foodie who seeks out new kitchen gadgets and delicious recipes to serve every food desire for Judith, as well as family and friends.

Judith is a music therapist, violinist, author/speaker & CEO at themusic4life.com, who seeks to serve through keynotes, webinars and telehealth, with constant gratitude for her protector, husband Dennis, her chef extraordinaire.

www.ingramcontent.com/pod-product-compliance
Lightning Source LLC
Chambersburg PA
CBHW042330150426
43194CB00001B/5